"Teachers, get ready to unlearn everything you think you know about health in schools. In *Ditching Weight Stigma and Anti-Fat Bias at School*, Cait O'Connor skillfully breaks down misinformation about health, size, food, and weight and gives teachers practical strategies to put their understanding into action. O'Connor makes the case that these topics are not just the responsibility of the health teacher, PE teacher, or school nurse, but a shared responsibility among everyone in a young person's life. You'll finish the book fired up to make change."

Alex Shevrin Venet, *author of* Equity Centered Trauma Informed Education *and* Becoming an Everyday Changemaker

"As someone who considers myself both a liberatory educator and a body-neutral teacher, parent, and human, *Ditching Weight Stigma and Anti-Fat Bias at School* exposes how much farther we all must go in evaluating how and what we teach about bodies. The book argues that anti-fat bias is so ingrained in our society, it's often hidden in the margins of curriculum and if we aren't actively fighting it, we're causing harm. Students deserve better, and this book is an explication on how to move ourselves and our schools forward. O'Connor's work is a rare gem that is thoughtful, accessible, and actionable from the first chapter, and I'm inspired to continue my own personal and professional journey against anti-fatness and liberation through the lens of this book. It's a must-read ASAP."

Chanea Bond, *literacy educator and scholar*

Ditching Weight Stigma and Anti-Fat Bias at School

Learn how anti-fat bias, weight stigma, and fatphobia show up in P-12 educational spaces and how that bias impacts the learners, educators, and communities where it happens.

In this important book, author Cait O'Connor reveals common problems with anti-fatness toward students in the classroom, in the curriculum, across subject areas, in the cafeteria, and after school. She also discusses anti-fatness toward teachers and staff. Throughout, she helps educators reflect on these issues and offers concrete solutions and equity fixes.

No matter what grade or subject you teach, you will benefit from the book's insightful research and practical strategies, and you'll come away prepared to help create a more equitable, stigma-free learning environment for all constituents.

Cait O'Connor (@JustTeachingELA) is an eighth-grade English/ENL teacher in Larchmont, New York. She is also a middle school American Sign Language Club advisor, mental health peer advocate, and an advocate for LGBTQIA+ youth, size inclusivity, peer-community engagement, and disability justice.

Equity and Social Justice in Education Series

Paul C. Gorski, Series Editor

Routledge's Equity and Social Justice in Education series is a publishing home for books that apply critical and transformative equity and social justice theories to the work of on-the-ground educators. Books in the series describe meaningful solutions to the racism, white supremacy, economic injustice, sexism, heterosexism, transphobia, ableism, neoliberalism, and other oppressive conditions that pervade schools and school districts.

Promoting Equitable Math Instruction
Exploring Elementary Teachers' Stories
Monica L. Gonzalez and Alesia Mickle Moldavan

The Social and Emotional Core of Equity Leadership
A Guide for Driving Change in Schools
Gianna Cassetta

Creating Inclusive Classrooms for Muslim Students
A Practical Guide for Teachers
Noor Ali

Teaching Environmental Justice in the Elementary Classroom
Entry Points for Equity Across the K-5 Curriculum
Kimi Waite

Ditching Weight Stigma and Anti-Fat Bias at School
Big and Small Equity Fixes for Educators
Cait O'Connor

Social Studies for a Better World
A Guide for Secondary Educators
Delandrea Hall, Katy Swalwell, and Noreen Naseem Rodríguez

Ditching Weight Stigma and Anti-Fat Bias at School

Big and Small Equity Fixes for Educators

Cait O'Connor

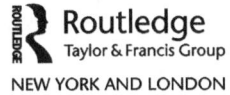

Routledge
Taylor & Francis Group

NEW YORK AND LONDON

Designed cover image: Getty Images

First published 2026
by Routledge
605 Third Avenue, New York, NY 10158

and by Routledge
4 Park Square, Milton Park, Abingdon, Oxon, OX14 4RN

Routledge is an imprint of the Taylor & Francis Group, an informa business

For Product Safety Concerns and Information please contact our EU representative GPSR@taylorandfrancis.com. Taylor & Francis Verlag GmbH, Kaufingerstraße 24, 80331 München, Germany.

ISBN: 978-1-032-87031-1 (pbk)
ISBN: 978-1-003-53414-3 (ebk)

DOI: 10.4324/9781003534143

Typeset in Palatino
by codeMantra

For my younger self

Contents

Acknowledgments

This book wouldn't have been possible without the inquiry and equity-minded support of Paul Gorski, editor of the *Equity and Social Justice in Education* series; or without shout-outs on social media from my friends Alex Shevrin Venet and Emily Zien. I am ever grateful to my best friend and best thought partner, Holly Spinelli, for encouraging me to write big and keep writing. I also want to thank Kayla Stansberry, Mikey Mercedes, educators Joana Munson, Adrienne Brandenberg, Drew Miller, Liz Browne, Aisha Atkinson, Chanea Bond, Abby Rose Morris, and my dear friend and co-builder Dr. Bilal Polson for your interviews. Big thanks to those whose own scholarship inspired me to write this book: Dr. Gholdy Muhammad, Cole Kazdin, Virginia Sole-Smith, Dr. Taylor Arnold, Shana Minei Spence, Dr. Bettina Love, Angie Manfredi, Esther Rothblum, Sondra Solovay, Aubrey Gordon, Paul Campos, Dr. Psyche Williams-Forson, Marilyn Wann, Carrie Safron, and Dillon Landi. To my editor Lauren Davis, thank you for answering all my questions, pushing me to write, and for (serendipitously!) living in the same zip code. To Hannah Sroka, for offering me guidance and always answering my emails. To my partner Mike and my dog Rocket, for all the time you spent going for walks without me and playing video games so I could write.

Meet the Author

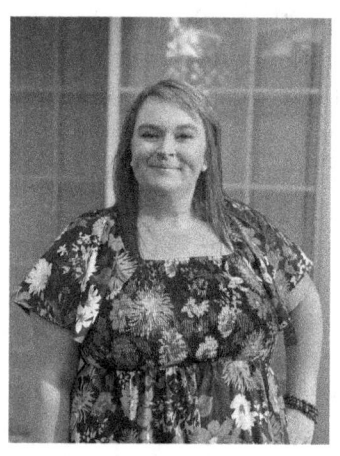

Cait O'Connor (she/her) is a middle school English Language Arts teacher in Westchester County, New York. She has taught middle school for five years and has been an educator for nine. She is also an avid reader, mental health peer advocate, hiker, and a dog mom. In 2020, Cait developed the Ditching Diet Culture at School digital library, a resource for educators, students, and parents on combating weight stigma. She has been published in journals like *Language Arts, English Journal*, and *English Leadership Quarterly*. In addition to presenting at various conferences in the United States about social justice, equity, inclusion, anti-fat bias, eating disorders, and body image, Cait was chosen as the National Council of Teachers of English 2023 Outstanding Middle Level Educator.

I

Press Play

In this part of the book, we will start the journey of unearthing anti-fat bias together. Along the way, we will encounter some ways to "remix" your thinking about anti-fat bias; but the first part of this book will be dedicated to seeing, hearing, and sensing things differently, so we can become aware of the inequities of fatphobia in all the parts of a school day.

DOI: 10.4324/9781003534143-1

1

Introduction

When I began my teaching career in 2017, it was also the same year I was aiming to find recovery and peace from a lifetime struggle against my body and food. As my positive body image increased, so did my weight.

Like many people in America, the message that "fat" was a synonym for "unhealthy," for "bad," for "lazy"; and that "fattening" foods were "bad," too – was on repeat. When I became an educator, social justice and impacting the world to make it more equitable and fair for all were top of mind. But it was this journey with my own body image that added anti-fat bias to the list of things that I noticed were visibly, tangibly inequitable about school – so I sought to change them. What led me there were hours of podcasts about recovery and body image, learning to love movement, and remixing my relationship to myself.

It felt impossible at first. After completing my undergraduate work, I worked as a preschool teacher – and trying to re-find a sense of positive body image while serving endless snacks to four year olds was an absolute nightmare. When I finally was called to start substitute teaching in a public school, so much diet talk surrounded me. I began wearing headphones and eating lunch alone just to avoid it. One afternoon between free periods, I read Lindo Bacon & Lucy Aphramour's *Body Respect: What Conventional*

DOI: 10.4324/9781003534143-2

Health Books Get Wrong, Leave Out, and Just Plain Fail to Understand about Weight, and a coworker asked me to explain what it was about. I talked about the social determinants of health, and how they were more closely related to a person's genetic and social propensity toward fatness than their individual behavior. They just laughed at what they felt was the ridiculousness of such a thought; how could being fat be anything *but* a fat person's own fault?

As I paid more attention to the ways we talked about food, weight, bodies, and people in society in general, I learned quickly – that fatphobia, healthism, size discrimination, and weight stigma – like many other forms of oppression – are initiated, acted out, and perpetuated at school.

Of course, I knew this as a student as early as second grade, living in a body experiencing her parents' divorce and navigating a relationship with myself and food at the same time. I paid careful attention to the ways that bodies were policed, talked about, shamed, and degraded by adults, and my friends and classmates. Like any other kid trying to dodge being the target, I probably (definitely) perpetuated and internalized some of that body negative messaging myself. I was a student during the era of Britney Spears, *Seventeen* magazine, and the tail end of when people still actually watched music videos on TV. When I became a teacher, I noted the pervasiveness of fatphobia (or, what Aubrey Gordon reframed as not a fear of fatness, but a hatred of it – anti-fatness)[1] not just between teachers in the faculty room, but in classrooms, at shared mealtimes, and even in curriculum. And, I thought – if I find this triggering as an adult, I can't imagine the harm it's doing to students and kids.

Whenever I've done professional development for educators, they've always given me the feedback that after our work together uncovering anti-fatness: "now it's everywhere – I can't unsee it." In our endeavor to create more equitable spaces for all students so they can thrive, that is the ultimate goal. As someone who associates music with their strongest memories – good and bad – I suppose, just like the bad things we've picked up about weight and body image, the inability to "unsee" weight stigma once we know it's there, is a pesky song stuck in our heads. At the core of our work are three actions: we will hit "play": that is, uncover anti-fat bias so that we can see it, see it so that we can pause it, and pause it so that we can create a new song – a remix of all the things we know, think we know, and thought we believed. Seeing, I find, comes with learning; but changing often bears the mammoth task of unlearning. I hope that what's ahead will illuminate anti-fat bias and weight stigma in our everyday educational system so that we can "hit pause" and start doing the work of changing it for the better – for our students, *and* for ourselves. Along the way, you will see the "B Sides" and "big moves": large and small pauses along the way meant to make you think on the journey – and in them, you will find tangible, doable, everyday actions to change and shift the ways your school shows up to make teaching and learning for people in larger bodies in your community.

It doesn't matter what content you teach or what grade you teach in; this is all of our work. If, like me, you are looking to stop anti-fatness at school or are looking for ways to illuminate it so that you *can* stop it – this book is for you. If you believe, like me, that each student deserves unrestricted, unconditional access to their learning, access to empathy and love, and to their understanding of themselves, this book is for you. Each of us in the education system has the power to notice the inequities of anti-fat bias, healthism, sizeism, and weight stigma so that we can create more just and equitable schools for all, and so that fat students, and *all* students, can learn and fat teachers, and *all* teachers, can teach. Weight bias, through its long and complicated history, remains alive despite something we can fix – a failure to see people as who they are, and difficulty forming relationships with them. My friend Alex Shevrin Venet, a changemaker, teacher, and expert on trauma-informed education, frequently reminds me through her work that learning is about relationships. Our learning spaces must teach students to live in harmony with our intersections, our differences and our entire *selves* – and that includes our bodies. We cannot expect to teach, or expect our students to learn – if they are not embodying the learning journey.

We'll start by defining some terms I've used so far to clarify their use throughout the text.

Anti-fat bias: Aubrey Gordon describes anti-fat bias as "an umbrella term used...to describe the attitudes, behaviors, and social systems that exclude, marginalize, underserve, and oppress fat bodies."[2] I would add that anti-fat bias harms fat bodies in this way, and morally and materially injures the *people* in those bodies.

Healthism: healthism is the idea that being "healthy" is morally superior or places people with no adverse health conditions on a moral high ground over those who don't. It is often used to perpetuate the "as long as you're healthy" fallacy that accompanies fat people and fat bodies, as if they owe proof of health to justify the way they look.

Sizeism: discrimination based on size, which becomes steeper the more fat a person is, or, conversely, the less thin privilege they have. For example, I do not need to buy two seats on a plane and am often read as someone who can shop for straight-sized clothing. I can shop in most stores, even if only in just a section, rather than ordering my clothes online or having them custom made.

Healthism and sizeism are a function of weight stigma, or the perception that fatness is morally, culturally, and socially inferior. Andrew Pickett & George Cunningham at Texas A&M University (2016)[3] state that "stigma separates individuals into distinct categories, each receiving differing levels of socio-political and cultural power based on group affiliation" – in other words, the thin/fat dichotomy is also the in/out group dichotomy.

Diet culture: the systemic and societal phenomenon that values thinness, and thin bodies, over all others, and promotes the use of often restrictive dieting as a means for becoming thin, no matter the cost. It is a phenomenon that has been promulgated by various industries, especially in the global North and the United States.

Thin privilege: an unearned series of accommodations or pathways granted to people who are straight-sized; things they do not have to think about in order to access a space, wear certain clothing, go certain places, get certain jobs because of the size or perceived size of their body.

A word on thin privilege and fat (social) identity: within fatness, there are varying degrees of privilege and marginalization. The following terms were coined by Ash from The Fat Lip Podcast, and are generally used in fat scholarship and fat studies. For instance, I am in a "mid fat" body; I wear a 2X–3X and can fit in most seats without accommodation, and though limited to a small section of the store, can shop at many retail stores for clothes. Someone smaller than me may identify or be identified as "small fat," and have these same or even more privileges, such as passing for thin and gaining more access. Folks who are larger than me, ranging from what is called large fat to superfat to infinifat, have less access to the things mentioned above because of their size.

Straight sized: anyone who does not need to shop in the "plus sized" section of a clothing store, who fits into most spaces without accommodation or assistance.

Additionally, note I use the word **fat** as a neutral descriptor throughout this text. It has a history of being used pejoratively that we will unpack at various points throughout the book, and interrogating the negative charge of this word is paramount to being able to access this work. If this is a struggle for you, be patient with yourself. If you find yourself flinching while reading or saying the word "fat" the first few times you see it or try to say it neutrally, note that this is a cultural and deeply rooted belief surfacing, and give yourself some grace. I honor (and know from experience) that this word has been used to bully, scapegoat, target, and harm different bodies. The words "obese" and "overweight" will be placed in quotations as often as possible except when quoted, because it is a medical term used to refer to fat people that now is ubiquitous and used in tandem with weight stigma. "Overweight" is not a synonym or a euphemism for fat, as it is often used – it is a term that pathologizes fat bodies and fat people to create pity around their "condition." Fat people do not need pity; we need freedom from weight stigma, diet culture, and bias – in the doctor's office, at school, and beyond. I hope that in healing your relationship to diet culture and body size, you will see, and use, the word fat as a "descriptor, not a discriminator," as Marilyn Wann once said.

I also hope that these definitions, as well as the rest of this book, aids you in reimagining schools in a fat-positive context. Throughout this book, we will focus on these principles for achieving fat positive, sustained equity for all: see anti-fatness, stop-anti-fatness, promote liberation, embodied learning, and body love.

RUN IT BACK: Reflecting on Your Practice

♦ *What do you need to get started on the journey to fat positive equity?*

♦ *What biases about fat people or health did you learn on your journey? Where did you learn them?*

♦ *What is your plan of action for unlearning, so you can be a more equitable educator and colleague for students and faculty in larger bodies?*

2

Facing the Music
Seeing Anti-Fat Bias as a Problem

Anti-fatness is everywhere, including schools.

As with any in/equity issue happening in a system, those within first have to see that it's happening in order to stop it from happening. Once we see and illuminate the problem, stopping the problem, or at least minimizing the harm that the inequity is doing to those who feel it the deepest, is our collective responsibility. Ending weight stigma so that students can experience fully embodied joy and justice at school is our collective responsibility.

From there, we can go from minimizing harm to creating environments that are, ideally, free of anti-fat harm. As author and campaigner Molly Forbes puts it in her book *Body Happy Kids: How to Help Children and Teens Love the Skin They're in*, "It stands to reason that a child or adolescent who is thinking about their body or outward appearance has less room in their head for phonics or improper fractions or whatever they're doing in class that day."[4] The need for spaces free of weight stigma, healthism, sizeism, and where inclusion is not only a stated value, but a felt, intrinsic value, has a direct relationship with equity. It is also a practice we must adopt, value, and sustain from an institutional level.

DOI: 10.4324/9781003534143-3

It isn't just an oversight that anti-fat bias is not included in our understanding of diversity, equity, inclusion, and belonging at school; it is an issue of justice. Anti-fat bias is ubiquitous, and hurts all of us; and it's an important paradigm to interrogate and address, especially given the historical and tangible intersections that anti-fat bias has with racism, classism, queerphobia, transphobia, and sexism.

Diversity, equity, inclusion, and belonging efforts that have found their way into schools often do not fully address the harm that is anti-fat bias, diet culture, or weight stigma. The educational system has perpetuated a body image crisis beginning as early as preschool. This calls for an interrogation of the problem of the epidemic and its framing: "If you think about how much of an impact body image anxiety has, the mental health capacities on young people and the way it prevents them from doing other things – to study, to focus, to want to speak out on important issues – if this was a new drug or some video games making our kids so unable to do things and eating into their time, we would be acting on it as a public health issue," stated Heather Widdows, a professor of philosophy at the University of Birmingham.[4]

Education has been the playground for various health initiatives like BMI report cards and campaigns like *Let's Move!* to address an "epidemic" of "obesity," all in the name of health.[2]

What if we, as a culture, reframed the real crisis as not the act of being fat, but understood the "war on obesity" as a "war on fat *people*"? And what if we responded to the body image crisis with compassion, justice, care, and respect?

Question the Built Environment, Not the Body

A lot of what makes up anti-fat bias is the false belief that fat is a changeable trait, and a matter of personal responsibility and willpower. Various industries perpetuate this belief, with a vested interest in keeping our self-esteem low and our internal shame meter (and their profits) high. Individuals are influenced by their environments, and this includes their overall health. Sometimes, environments may act as a stressor, exerting unhealthful influence on mood, performance, and physiology.[5] School environments where weight stigma is allowed can facilitate both implicit and explicit weight bias, teasing, and become a source of trauma and stress for students.

Challenging the idea that fat is unhealthy, disgusting, or inherently inferior is not popular or easy; heck, most times it isn't even politically neutral. As such, many approaches to challenging anti-fat bias have started, and ended, with the premise that epigenetics, social determinants, and other factors mean that we should be nicer to fat kids because "they can't help it." I'm going to challenge this notion and replace it with the idea that we should be nicer to fat kids because they are HUMAN. This also requires educators and anyone working in the context of a school to see fat kids/folks as a group of people with an identity that is both a non-issue and limited by their built environment in a multitude of ways: body violence, microaggressions, oppressive structures, barriers to access, etc. These barriers highlight our responsibility as educators and changemakers to transform the built environment...not the kids. What if we taught children about health in a way that is just as differentiated, diverse, and intersectional as they are? What if we could reimagine the school day, the school building, and the lives of students and teachers so that our efforts at belonging send the message that fat bodies matter, so all bodies matter? What we have now is a system that enables the bullying, discrimination, and declining academic outcomes of students in larger bodies – and makes school traumatic for them in the process. Not only does the current paradigm create body-based trauma for fat kids; it creates a false sense of moral superiority and inherited, socialized anti-fat bias in thin ones. Fatphobia brings about trauma that we all collectively struggle with, whether or not we know it – a form of silent or implicit trauma that, like sexism and racism, "has to do with a violation of an entire demographic of people via cultural structures."[6] And while everyone lives and breathes diet culture, not everyone knows and lives the reality of anti-fatness.

Virginia Sole-Smith, in her essay "What Thin Kids Need to Learn About Fatphobia," states:

> If we don't talk about these different forms of oppression, the kids who aren't victims of said oppression are more likely to become perpetrators. They can see that the world treats Black people and fat people and otherwise marginalized people worse than it treats white, thin, privileged people.[7]

Children learn about body bias as early as age three, and negative attitudes toward body size and higher-weight people reach back into the 1960s.[8] If kids cannot see anti-fat bias, that is, if they become "body-blind," they learn that the thin privilege they have makes them somehow innately, naturally better than the people who don't have it.

In her 2022 *Edutopia* article, Paige Tutt writes:

> Within schools, the implications are both moral and practical. As more and more students grow up with the all-consuming feeling that something is wrong with the body they occupy, the consequences can range from toxic environments that marginalize the physically nonconforming to the prospect of classrooms full of students so anxious about how they look that learning itself is compromised.[9]

Two different studies, done in 2011 and 2016 respectively, report that among adolescents, weight-based bullying is the most common type of bullying they encounter at school – more than bullying based on disability, race, religion, gender, or other identity factors. In the 2011 study, the researchers found that at least 84 percent of participants observed overweight students being teased "in a mean way and teased during physical activities," and 65–77 percent of students observed overweight and obese peers "being ignored, avoided, excluded from social activities."[10] Teachers and staff are aware of it, too. In a 2011 study of over 5,000 American educators and school professionals, weight-based bullying was seen to be a larger problem than bullying based on sex, race, sexual orientation, or disability. In a U.S. survey of 918 parents, "weight was perceived to be the most common reason youth were bullied, and parents' views remained consistent regardless of their own child's weight status"[11]

The curve of discrimination experiences gets even steeper for students who are multi-marginalized; that is, kids who are fat and poor, fat and LGBTQIA+, and fat and BIPOC experience even more bullying at school than their peers who have some level of racial, cisgender, or socioeconomic privilege, even the ones who are higher weight.[12]

These findings make clear why weight and size diversity awareness should happen earlier in a child's life than school – because they're being made aware of whose bodies are deserving of dignity and whose are deserving of derision well before then. Kids who don't experience anti-fat bias happening at/to/around them need critical thinking about body size and image in order to build knowledge, awareness, and empathy. As they grow into school-aged students and then into adulthood, the adverse mental health effects and school-based trauma they remember only increase the longer we allow fatphobia to fester. In the next chapter, we will discuss how these mental health impacts and the material harm of bullying for fat kids can impact their academic and social outcomes during, and after, the school day.

Where Does Fat Hate Originate?

In order to understand how we got here, we must first understand how various industries have worked together to codify the idea that fat = bad, and the belief that that is an objective thought; rather than one rooted in bias from various medical, statistical, and individual opinions that became the sentiment of an entire population. In *You Have the Right to Remain Fat*, Virgie Tovar states powerfully that "fatphobia creates an environment of hostility toward larger-bodied people [and] promotes a pathological relationship to food and movement"[13] which, inevitably, results in the spirit murder[14] from an early age: kids learn to hate their bodies, and schools have in many cases made that dynamic worse. Tovar states: "Most people are raised to believe myriad bigoted beliefs about fat inferiority and see this fictional creation as a natural truth. They don't see these beliefs as political, cultural, or particularly problematic. They often don't even know they have these feelings."[15] I have found this to be true as an educator who sees these attitudes sold as "health" and missing altogether from conversations about diversity, equity, inclusion, belonging, and justice.

The adage often circulated among school professionals about any form of discrimination or prejudiced attitudes about a specific group is that "hate starts at home." But this sentiment often reduces the learning of prejudice to parents and passes down attitudes of privilege and supremacy without question; without examining the culture that made it possible for those attitudes to take shape and flourish. Anti-fat bias may begin in the doctor's office, and be transferred to parents, before making its way to the playground. But it's also echoed in the cafeteria, in the classroom, and reverberates throughout faculty lounges, too. Our collective responsibility to address bullying cannot begin and end with "be kind," especially if the mixed messaging of "health" comes with a side of "equals thinness" at every turn in a child's education.

Numerous studies reveal that a common source of weight stigma is within the family.[9] The idea that "hate starts at home" does not let schools off the hook for their history of upholding inequities and biases. This includes bias and prejudice toward people because of their size, race, class, gender, orientation, or other identity factors. Let's look at some of the ways that anti-fat hate (and simultaneously, racism, ableism, and classism) has been codified into attitude, practice, policy, and even standards of care.

A Belgian social researcher named Adolphe Quetelet, who sought in the 1830s to use mathematics to quantify the "ideal man." Thus, he invented a widely used ratio in determining health.[16] His equation worked like this: multiply a person's weight in kilograms by their height in centimeters, squared, and the percentage measures the person up to his ideal or "average."

In the mid-20th century, prominent researcher Ancel Keys sought to influence the medical industry and find a "more effective" measure of weight.[17] He saw the Quetelet Index as "not fully satisfactory," so he sought to rebrand the way we measured body composition. Keys transformed Quetelet's Index into body mass index, or BMI, and led a study of over 7,500 men from different, but mostly white, countries – Finland, the United States, Italy, Japan, and South Africa (countries with radically different relationships to their environment and epidemiology). At the end, the published study also excluded its own findings about Black South African men, because it felt that they "could not be a representative sample of all [Black] men in Cape Province, let alone [Black] men in general." During the time of Keys' research, BMI only "diagnosed" "obesity" accurately about 50 percent of the time.[17] BMI also does not discriminate between muscle and fat when calculating a person's mass, and when it comes to using it as a measure of health for kids, "BMI doesn't take into consideration changes in growth patterns" or the differing body composition overall that children have from adults.[17] The study and its subsequent implications in the medical industry, however, were well on their way to becoming the nexus for conflating weight and health, despite this acknowledged flaw and the fact that it did not include women or other evolutionary factors in its findings.

Another problem with using BMI to evaluate children: Quetelet didn't study anyone except white, able-bodied European men who were eligible for military service, and he never intended to. In fact, weight was not considered even a primary or independent indicator of health until the 19th century, when insurance companies like MetLife and the mathematicians who worked for them such as Louis Dublin, began to use Quetelet's index to compile weight and height charts to determine how much to charge life insurance policy holders.[17, 16]

Though later in his career he criticized the origins of the MetLife weight/height charts and the very idea of "ideal" or "desirable" weight as "armchair concoctions," he still maintained that "obesity" [was] "unsightly," "disgusting," and "repugnant." He admitted in later statements that "obesity" did not necessarily cause heart disease, [but] it was nevertheless, in his view, "ugly."[16]

Keys' views were absorbed into the medical community, which were transmitted swiftly into our society at large, paving the way for pharmaceutical industries to look for ways to profit off the idea that losing weight meant "getting healthy" and promising that they had the solution. The diet industry, as we know it today, also took shape around this narrative that people *had* to lose weight "for their health." Despite evidence that heart disease and other illnesses we have stereotyped as "fat people illnesses" today were not *caused* by high weight, and no evidence that these diseases occur any less frequently in thin people – it is the fear that is used to keep people in perpetual pursuit of weight loss.[2, 17, 16]

Negative attitudes toward fatness and fat people can also be intergenerational and inherited. About the process of writing her book *Fat Talk: Parenting in the Age of Diet Culture*, Virginia Sole-Smith states,

> It really became clear to me that people were saying "I want my kid to have a good relationship with food. I want them to love their body. I don't want them to get an eating disorder. But I don't want them to be fat." And we can't have it both ways.[18]

In her book, Sole-Smith interviews various families about the role of diet culture in their lives; some of whom went to extreme measures to curtail their kids' eating habits, like putting their favorite foods in a lockbox. Still others, even after reporting the negative impacts of diet culture, reported later that they were bringing their child to a weight loss clinic.[18]

The grip that diet culture has on parents, even when they know of the harm it causes, reveals so much about the deep roots of the belief that fat is undesirable and should be avoided. Even well-meaning parents try to blunt the word fat with euphemisms; but as fat activist Marilyn Wann once said, "large, big-boned, overweight, chubby, voluptuous, plump, and obese are all synonyms for fear."[19]

While most people think of bullying as the source of weight stigma, it is merely a strand in this more complicated web.

Weight stigma and the myth that being mean to fat people is somehow "motivating" is what causes bullying. Many of these attitudes start in the doctor's office and circulate around the dinner table before finding their way into schools. In a research letter published in the *Journal of American Medicine Pediatrics* in 2014, weight stigma researchers Jeffrey Hunger and A. Janet Tomiyama note that "stigma processes can begin when an individual experiences weight labeling. By labeling someone as overweight, the negative stereotypes, status loss, and mistreatment associated with this label may now be applicable to the individual."[20] That is to say, it's not the fact of being fat that causes weight stigma, shame, and oppression; but what we are supposed to think it *means* about a person; about their status, their willpower, their moral character, and even their intelligence. After all, if they were intelligent and could control themselves, how could they look like *that*? Hunger and Tomiyama's research also found that being labeled "too fat" in childhood or adolescence was associated with higher odds of having a BMI in the "obese" category nearly a decade later. So, weight *stigma* is actually known to turn children, whether or not they are fat, into fat adults.

Even with the good intentions of parents and caretakers in these food-limiting (and fat-controlling) behaviors being about "wellness," they are largely rooted more in a fear that stems from social pressure.

> Given the enormous social pressure to lose weight, one might suppose there is clear and overwhelming evidence of the risks of obesity and the benefits of weight loss. Unfortunately, the data linking overweight and death, as well as the data showing the beneficial effects of weight loss are limited, fragmentary, and often ambiguous.[21]

The parenting piece of the social pressure to stay thin (and help kids stay thin) comes from the way we view, police and access parents and caregivers. School systems are entangled with other systems of child welfare and wellness, and sometimes, a child's weight has been cause for concern and even removal of a child from the care of their parents who love them. In the United States and the UK there are examples of children who have been placed in foster care or with other family members for the simple fact of their being "too fat."[9, 18]

Most parents seek, and internalize, diet culture and anti-fat bias from a place of good intentions, from being told that it's "for their child's health." After all, isn't that the same message they were given as children, and their parents received as children? What Marilyn Wann said in 1998 still rings true today:

> Fat children get extra lessons when their parents – with the best of intentions – put them on diets. The parents don't want their children to be teased. They don't want their children to have health problems. The child doesn't see a diet that way. All the fat child knows is that she gets teased at school for being fat, and instead of her parents protecting her from that trauma, they basically agree with her bullies and take away her food. Now the child is unhappy AND hungry. The message children get from such parental intervention is this: "If you're fat, there's something wrong with you. We'd love you more if you were thinner."[19]

It makes sense that the intergenerational (and sometimes self-contradicting) messaging of anti-fat bias is a few decades deep, given its passing down from the fathers of early eugenics to researchers to medical professionals, whose relationship with the pharmaceutical industry (and its younger sibling, the diet industry) is unmistakable and ubiquitous. As Virgie Tovar points out in her book,

> Because of the way fat people are positioned in our culture, people learn to fear becoming fat. They are afraid of discrimination and hatred. It is normal to feel afraid of people hating you. It is not normal for people to hate anyone based on how much they weigh.[15]

The current generation's fraught relationship with food and body may also have roots in wartime food rationing bestowed upon their grandparents and great-grandparents, in which mixed messages about food waste, civic duty, and beauty standards clashed in the minds of the American psyche. As a child of divorced parents, different food rules, recipes, eating times, activity expectations, body types, and projections of body image made navigating this so deeply confusing.

In *Fat Talk*, Virginia Sole-Smith outlines the contradicting lessons in these kinds of messages to kids, which start at home – and make their way to school in different iterations. "The belief that children should eat any food put in front of them, without complaint, doesn't allow for much individuality of preference. And worse, it frames eating as a moral and behavioral issue," she elaborates, saying

> No matter what motivation drives it, demanding clean plates is, at its core, a lesson in control. It's a parent saying to their child – I know what's best for your body. You need to put this in your body – even though you don't want to – because I said you should.[18]

The converse of the "clean plate" effect, at least for me, was that it messed with my own hunger and fullness cues in this way and other ways. I felt guilty for not eating foods I didn't want, didn't like, or had had enough of. As I tried to balance what foods, and how much of them, I wanted, the opposite of the coin was said in my direction more frequently – are you *really* going to eat all of *that*?

The message I received was the same as Sole-Smith described: *you don't know what amount of food is best for you, even though your body is trying to tell you you're hungry; listen to our feedback instead.* Fat kids hear this message all the time, as if their bodies are a minefield and they are one bad choice away from a health crisis. And under the intention and assumption of "protecting" them, their parents teach them to eat furtively, binge privately, and loathe themselves perpetually. "There is a straight line for many people from these kinds of high pressure dinner tables to allow diet culture to control how and what they eat. And that is especially true when 'clean your plate' is mixed together with 'but don't get fat.'"[18]

One standout memory for me was at an after-school program I attended in elementary school, which provided us snacks before we started our homework. Given that at my elementary school, lunch was at 11 o'clock in the morning and I had gotten to after-care by 3:45, it made sense that I was hungry after four hours without a meal as a growing seven year old – and a plate of four Saltine crackers and some juice was just not going to cut it. So I asked for seconds.

"It's like your hobby is eating. You do not stop!" laughed the teacher, with other kids joining in to make fun of me for the crime of my hunger. That was my first lesson in learning that actually, other people knew my body better than I did.

In her 2019 essay for *SELF*, Aubrey Gordon writes:

> Growing up as a fat kid meant hearing judgments, derision and outright revulsion of fat bodies at every turn: from family, friends, doctors, media, teachers. And at the center of it all were bodies like mine: the bodies of fat kids. I was a sixth grader, bare in a spotlight, defined by her insufficiency.[22]

Gordon, who is white and identifies as fat and queer, has contributed much to the conversation about anti-fat bias and the research that is continually used to do harm to fat people. Like Gordon, people in my life knew my body better than me. But, ironically, despite years of binging and restricting, I evaded intervention as long as that body remained a thin one.

> **Quick Tip**
>
> *Practice saying the word fat without any negative connotation. Model it for your thin peers and friends, especially if you are in a thin body.*

Schools Help Shape the Narrative

School-aged children using weight control as an indirect method for maintaining social clout (or minimally, just maintaining invisibility and avoiding bullying) is a product of the myths that weight is something we have total control over and that thinness is more desirable. But what about when the school *itself* reinforces this dynamic of body shame, thin superiority, and anti-fat bias?

When I was a student, we learned about nutrition largely from our health teacher, always in the context of the ever-evolving food pyramid and BMI. I don't remember having to do weigh-ins (thankfully) at all, let alone publicly, but that did not stop the shaming microaggressions from being parceled into curriculum.

I went home and worked out even after practice, sometimes for hours, using, of all things, the Wii Fit, and tabulating my BMI and basal metabolic rate (BMR) and every calorie burned into a spreadsheet while blasting "Misery Business" by Paramore and doing crunches into the hundreds. I weighed myself nearly every morning, and attached these numbers, compulsively calculated and carefully sweat out, to my worth.

The thing is, when I was performing all these insane tasks to avoid living in a fat body, I was a thin kid who ran cross-country and track on top of regularly (compulsively) exercising. But my exercise wasn't driven by a love of movement – it was driven by a fear of fat. I developed eating disorders across the spectrum, and oscillated back and forth between binging, restricting, and purging via exercise until well into college. I don't know if my body would be a fat body today if I hadn't taken it on this rollercoaster driven by fear, weight stigma, and media messaging that no amount of calorie deficit was good enough. And because I stayed thin for most of it, these behaviors went undetected by nearly everyone around me. It echoed my first experiences with food shaming, when assumptions were made about my hunger and I was told, by outside sources, what was best for my growing body; now, assumptions about my health, conflated with thinness, meant I could avoid any intervention for my problematic eating behaviors because my appearance did not reflect that of someone who ate a box of Triscuits in its entirety after a run, or seven 13-ounce jars of Nutella in a week between twice-a-day gym workouts – or what they thought the body of someone who did these things *should* look like.

Witnessing weight-based bullying at school impacts adolescents' perception of the importance of thinness, and has been linked to school-aged students experiencing "poorer body image, lower self-esteem, depressive symptoms, unhealthy weight and shape control behaviors, and muscle-enhancing behaviors,"[23] even if that bullying is not happening directly to them.

The message they are getting from weight-based bullying is that in order to avoid teasing, they should seek and maintain thinness by any means necessary. This myth purports a kind of victim-blaming that fat kids often hear: *If you want them to stop bullying you, then you should "just" lose weight.* It is particularly pervasive in the United States, "which," Jacqueline Weinstock and Michelle Krehbiel argue, "values self discipline and thinness." The same can be said of the ways we study fatness in relation to health: plenty of research validates the existence of weight stigma and the fact that weight stigma, not "obesity," leads to poor outcomes. But the answer is almost always to tell the fat person, if you don't want to experience stigma, discrimination, or social inferiority, *you* need to change. Weinstock and Krehbiel also say that "Unfortunately, this view of weight as controllable leads many to blame those who are fat for being fat, and thus treat fatness as an individual character flaw."[24] It tells kids that they will remain less likely to be targeted as long as they stay thin, or, at the very least, remain in proximity to or in pursuit of thinness. In a society where "people freely express prejudice against fat people," how are we supposed to support youth who face weight-based bullying when so many of our institutions promote it? Weinstock and Krehbiel assert that "The willingness to express prejudice against fat people is itself influenced by the tendency for weight to be seen as controllable."[24]

Are schools just unaware of how weight labeling causes weight stigma, and the effects of those fear and shame tactics are counter to their goal of "educating" American kids about health? The answer, I think, lies somewhere in the middle of all the places where various industries, like food marketing, form alliances with educational institutions, including ones that believe that weight can be controlled – and permanently sustained, through "lifestyle changes" (diets). It's the only way these contradicting messages about health and how they are packaged to students could make any sense. As it stands right now, schools are a place where kids in larger bodies are being made to wonder "what's wrong with *me*?" and we respond by effectively telling them, through too-small desks, stigmatizing curriculum, and shaming policy that they will have access to learning as soon as *they*, not their environments, make changes. In her book *Unearthing Joy*, Dr. Gholdy Muhammad says, "a school that is truly equitable embraces fairness and inclusion, and it responds to students' individual needs, providing structures, systems and practices that enable all students to reach their highest potential for personal and academic success."[25] In a school where fatphobia exists, and students who experience it are made responsible for not bringing it on themselves every time it happens to them, equity cannot, and does not, exist. She draws on the metaphor of curriculum design as a dress fitting – and the hands that design it are, outside of this metaphor, quite literally working to erase the identities of children in larger bodies. She says:

> When the creation does not fit a child, we say things such as "The child needs an intervention, and put the onus on the child and not the curriculum. Can you imagine if a designer created a gown for you, without your input, without learning about you, and when the day comes to try it on, it's too small – and you're told you need to go on a diet or gain weight? And you think, *but you never took my measurements.* That's what's happening in schools.[25]

In terms of size diversity and equity, this metaphor is literally happening to kids in schools – the onus being put on them to change the very bodies they live and learn in. We are handing them a curriculum that seeks to "intervene" in their corporeality if they are a certain size, and the forces of policy, money, and curriculum are tools used to send them messages that their bodies are wrong.

I talked with Mikey Mercedes (she/they), a public health researcher and co-host of the podcast *Unsolicited: Fatties Talk Back* about their experiences with these intersections in their own school experience. When we talked, Mikey shared a few anecdotes with me about their lived experience as a young, fat Black kid that were particularly striking.

One such anecdote was about the ways Mikey was weight labeled by a school counselor as early as second grade.

> These boys in my second grade class would giggle every time I shifted in my chair and I tried to talk to my teacher about it. I went to the school psych[ologist] and she was like, "Why do you think they're giggling at you?" and I said "I think it's because I'm too big for my chair."
>
> She wasn't quite weight loss counseling me, but she was telling me that sometimes when you're a bigger kid, kids that are smaller than you will make fun of you; and that it's not a good thing, but part of it is good because it should be motivation to be more active.
>
> I never spoke to anyone about anything weight or size related [at school] again after that.

Weight labeling that happens under the guise of being "motivational" assumes a lot about fat kids' health and makes them feel like their bodies, not their bullies, are the issue.

"When you live in a world where your body is pathological – when it is sick, diseased, unruly, malformed, or seen as inherently wrong, suddenly everybody is a doctor," Mikey said. "My school psych was not a healthcare provider, but she assumed a clinical gaze and decided I needed to be told that [weight-based bullying was a good thing] in order to become a less fat second grader." These kinds of conversations are examples of microaggressions and victim blaming.

Weight labeling and weight-based bullying are not unique to American schooling, however. In her study "Bon Bon Fatty Girl: A Qualitative Exploration of Weight Bias in Singapore," Maho Isono, Patti Lou Watkins, and Lee ee. Lian discuss research subject Melinda, who reported that her teacher drew a round face on the board that was supposed to be her, and she "subsequently thought of herself as stupid, clumsy and fat." Another teacher in the study, who was from Britain, detailed a story during which secondary schoolchildren were weighed publicly, and "the nurse communicated to one girl that she was 'so fat and lazy' and 'was doing nothing to help herself'." "The girl, by now in tears, pleaded that she ran to school everyday, but the nurse just wouldn't believe her."[26] This data illustrates that anti-fatness in school spaces is not unique to America, or even to the West; and that it can cross cultures and impact students at school on a global scale, asking them to justify themselves as "good," despite their fat, even in the face of bullying from adults charged with caring for them.

Weight stigma is pervasive among peers, teachers, and all members of school communities. Instead of teaching students they are less capable, what we should be teaching all kids is that all bodies have inherent dignity, worth, and value, and that their worth is not equal to their appearance, weight, or size. And we can do this by centering those at the margins and creating spaces that welcome them unconditionally so that they can learn.

Cultivating Respect

To date, 49 states have enacted anti-bullying laws, but only three states in the United States have anti-bullying laws that explicitly mention weight as a protected status – New York, New Hampshire, and Maine.[27] It is legal to discriminate against people based on weight in almost every country in the world at a national level, though states such as Michigan are enacting legislation making that discrimination illegal in spaces such as the workplace. This supports my own "bite-sized" research; in a survey taken in January 2024 of 39 users on X, 24 users reported that their school system does not have any measures or policies in place to address weight-based discrimination or bullying; ten said they were not sure; and only one answered yes.

Public support for anti-bullying laws to explicitly address bullying and discrimination against people because of their weight, perceived weight, or size is high in countries such as the United States, Iceland, Canada, and Australia – 75–96 percent of parents surveyed support an expansion of anti-bullying legislation to protect children from weight-based bullying.[11]

In the state of New York, there are laws on the books such as DASA (the Dignity for All Students Act), passed in 2011, which considers weight as a protected class as part of its legislation.[28] All teachers in the state are required to receive and even renew training in DASA as part of their licensing requirements.

Yet, New York is one of half of U.S. states which also requires schools to collect "Student Weight Status Data."[29] It has collected this data annually since 2010, and findings reveal students are in the BMI range "overweight" or "obese" most often in middle and high school, and in districts across the state that it considers "high needs," which can mean that families in that school system are of a lower socioeconomic status (SES) or that there are more BIPOC students and families living and attending school there – or a combination of the two.

> **Quick Tip**
>
> *If your school sends out BMI reporting notices, and you can do so, let caretakers and students know that it is their right to opt out of having this data collected.*

What New York's Student Weight Status Data does not address is that body mass index was never designed to measure the "health" of these communities where it reports as being highest in the first place. The ways that our curriculum and school systems are set up inevitably lead to exclusion and even physical and psychological bullying of fat kids, and a fear of weight gain among thin ones. What do we do when the curriculum itself is the bully?

Youth and Weight-Based Bullying

Research shows that "Adolescents with a BMI percentile in the healthy weight range were least likely to report weight-based teasing from family (47.5%) or peers (39.3%)."[30] This part of the study is unsurprising, because benefiting from thin privilege shields people somewhat from teasing, as long as they "fit the norm"; but it does not guarantee total evasion of soaking up, or being subject to, anti-fat bias.

The study also reported that cisgender boys and transgender girls experienced the least weight-based bullying from their family in the study, which reveals the ways that misogyny and cissexism (the privileging of cisgender people and bodies) place different expectations on boys, and even furthers this expectation and norm about body size, weight, and perception of size and weight into the realm of transmisogyny. Transgender girls aren't seen as "feminine" in a cissexist world; and this may point to the reasons they more carefully evade weight-shaming, especially if they are not fat to begin with. The researchers found that "Between 43% and 55% of gender minorities experienced weight-based teasing from peers, with the highest percentages reported by transgender boys (55.3%), transmasculine/non-binary adolescents (53.9%), and transfeminine/non-binary (52.6%) adolescents."[30]

Transgender boys and transmasculine adolescents may be subject to more weight-based teasing for the same misogynistic and transmisogynistic reasons, because fat is seen as effeminate, soft, and less likely to help them "pass." These assumptions and intersections of gender, transphobia, and anti-fat bias help serve the gender binary, and create less safety and belonging for trans and gender nonconforming students at school, and can even impact their attendance and educational outcomes. Additionally, trans and gender nonconforming students are more likely than their cisgender peers to develop eating disorders, because body dysmorphia can often accompany gender dysphoria.[31] It also reveals the prejudice of doctors about trans bodies and fat bodies, because their refusal to do top surgeries has even come packaged in the form of "not looking as good" on larger bodies. And doctors often do not even consider patients, regardless of age, for gender-affirming care unless they are below a certain BMI, furthering the stigma and isolation of transgender people and youth, especially ones who are fat.

Alex Gino, author of the middle-grade book *Melissa*, discusses their experiences being both fat and trans in Angie Manfredi's YA collection *The Other F Word: A Celebration of the Fat and Fierce*. In it, they write:

> The fat person who becomes thin is a cultural hero. They have defeated the demons of fat and sugar and sloth and receive accolades of moral triumph...but the trans person

who transitions is a burden. There are new names and pronouns to learn, mistakes not to make. Public questions of bathrooms and athletic competitions. We complicate the system by making the system visible.[32]

Gino's experience highlights the double standard of body autonomy that is not given to trans people, especially when those trans people are fat. Schools reinforce this system through the gender binary, bathrooms, locker rooms, athletics, ceremonies and rites of passage segregated by gender, etc. Gino continues, "The fat body that loses weight is conforming, where the fat body that takes hormones and/or has surgery is pushing conformity for the right to exist."[32] Either way, fat or trans and fat and trans kids are not playing to win, because school isn't made for them to. The design of the system asks for their conformity, of both size and gender, every day, in most aspects of their learning.

In recent years, increased cases of bullying and "bullycide" have led to the need for legislation to address anti-bullying efforts, and litigation following deaths by suicide of teens who are mercilessly bullied. Such was the case for seventeen-year-old Eric Mohat, who was called homophobic slurs by his peers during math class. The lawsuit cites a teacher who failed to intervene and parents who, aching from their son's loss, sought not compensation, but acknowledgement that their son had been, quite literally, bullied to death. His death in 2009 is one of thousands of cases brought to light of the horrors of bullying and the need for anti-bullying laws, especially ones that protect LGBTQIA+ youth.[33]

Following the death of Eric Mohat, and the national news stories of "bullycide" deaths of 13-year-old Seth Walsh, of 13-year-old Asher Brown, and Rutgers freshman Tyler Clementi, projects like It Gets Better launched in response to stop bullying, pass deterrent legislation, and support youth – and parents across the United States supported this passage as well as the use of litigation to protect students from bullying on the basis of identity. But, Puhl et al. found in their study that those interviewed showed more support for litigating bullying related to race and sexual orientation than weight.[11] Though most cases of bullying do not reach the point where litigation is needed, research points to the fact that everyone in a school community generally sees weight-based bullying as a problem. Still, parents support litigation on the basis of weight-based bullying less often than they do for suits that involve bullying based on race and other identity factors. This, perhaps, points back to the outdated idea that weight is controllable, and if you're not doing anything to get the target off your back, bullies have earned the right to do their worst. This makes the need for education against diet culture and size acceptance even more necessary. In *Fat! So?* Marilyn Wann says,

> We cannot expect individual fat kids to rise up courageously and silence their tormentors any more than we expect children of color to defend against racist comments all by themselves. Our opposition to fat hatred should be just as vehement, just as immediate, and just as certain as our opposition to racism.[19]

For some kids, the link between fatphobia and racism is played out on their bodies *by* the state. Such was the case for Anamarie Regino, a 90-pound three-year-old who was born in Albuquerque. For Anamarie, the hate did not start at home – but it instead tore her home apart. She was taken from her parents and placed into foster care because social services assumed her parents were neglecting her health. The state of New Mexico made racist assumptions about her Latinx family, citing her mother's presumed inability to speak English as a reason they perceived that the family did not know about health. Although they spoke English, raised their daughter in an English-speaking household, and regularly took Anamarie to the doctor; even as recently as three weeks before her removal from the home – the state separated Anamarie from her parents because she was fat.[18, 34]

In 1997, a British girl named Kelly Yeomans died by suicide in her home after facing relentless anti-fat bullying from her peers. She was 13. Boys from her school reportedly went to her house in Derby several nights in a row, throwing butter, margarine, cake, and dirt at her family home and yelling "smelly Kelly" to her through the window. Her parents suspected she was depressed, but did not realize it was serious enough that she would take her life. The margarine-throwing was the incident that led to her suicide – but she had endured three years of being called "fatty," having her lunch soiled at school, and having her school clothes tossed in the trash by bullies.[35]

Intersectional Inequalities

The admission that "obesity" has been found, even as far back as Ancel Keys' 1956 "Seven Countries Study" not to be a *cause* of heart disease, but to instead have correlation with it, is huge. Correlation and causation flaws drive so much of what we know (or think we know) about health, and how we translate what we think we know to kids in schools. We must interrogate these biases and their entanglement with various industries, including the ways we teach everything from health, science, literature, statistics, to media literacy.

In *What We Don't Talk About When We Talk About Fat*, Aubrey Gordon says, "According to studies published by the Endocrine Society, the BMI overestimates fatness and health risks for Black people. Meanwhile, according to the WHO, the BMI underestimates health risks for Asian communities, which may contribute to underdiagnosis of conditions such as heart disease, diabetes, and other illnesses."[17] Her book also describes a study that "details the ways in which people of color in a "healthy" BMI range are assumed not to be at risk for cardiovascular or pancreatic issues." This illustrates the flaws in relying on one measure, the BMI, as a predictor of health, and leaning on weight rather than epigenetics, family history, and cultural identity to tell us something about the health of our students and their families. Schools being used as a vehicle for the collection of this data, with no plan to address the social determinants of health that are related to it, puts schools, and the administrators and teachers who work for them, in a position to be purveyors of weight stigma and anti-fat bias against students and their families.

A longitudinal study conducted by Project EAT (Eating Among Teens) measured eating and weight-related variables in

4,746 adolescent boys and girls, as well as their experiences with weight-related teasing. The study found that

> Asian-American boys, black boys, and Asian-American girls reported lower prevalences of peer teasing than whites. Hispanic, Asian-American, and mixed/other girls reported higher prevalences of family weight teasing than did white girls. In nearly all racial/ethnic groups for all three teasing variables, obese adolescents were significantly more likely to report having been teased, compared to average-weight adolescents.[36]

The study also found that Black girls were "less bothered" by the weight-based teasing than their white female peers.

The supposition that white girls are "more bothered" by anti-fat bullying than Black girls is telling of the intersectional negative impacts of weight stigma, misogyny, and anti-Blackness. Whiteness and anti-fatness go hand-in-hand, because it has long been used as a way of justifying, even "scientifically," the superiority of white people, especially among white women. I don't think Black girls find fatphobia any less damaging or oppressive than their white counterparts; I think it speaks to the inherent white fragility that accompanies thinness. In fact, it's been studied and found that Black and Latine girls have better body image, but also larger bodies, than their white female peers; but initiatives designed by diet industries coupled with policy initiatives have dulled their confidence, in the name of "doing something about" their weight and size in the name of health.[37] To be Black and fat in a white supremacy culture are culturally synonymous with social inferiority, and thinness is how whiteness remains standing at the top of the social hierarchy. When it's said that fatphobia is the "last acceptable form of oppression," we must be quick to point out that we live in a society where oppressions like racism, gender-based violence, queerphobia, and ableism *in addition to* anti-fatness are the reality of many people globally.

Adolphe Quetelet, with his search for the "ideal man" or *l'homme moyenne*, inspired and eventually influenced Sir Francis

Galton, a cousin of Charles Darwin and the father of eugenics – to quantify that moral superiority into a "science."[17, 16] Black girls, and by extension, Black people, have never been part of "the ideal" of the "West"; and have had to bear the burden of multiple intersecting oppressions including anti-fatness. *In Fearing the Black Body: The Racial Origins of Fatphobia*, Sabrina Strings states that "the thin ideal has been used both to degrade Black women and discipline white women."[16] But the BMI isn't only flawed because it historically excluded Black people from its data gathering. It's flawed because it's been historically used as a measuring stick for people's health, which is equated to their worth and humanity, and used to justify the injustice perpetrated against them. The intersections between race, class, gender, and fat meet here, and school is no exception.

"There's something to be said about the damaging aspects of going to school or living in a place that has less weight diversity," says Mikey Mercedes.

> There is social, emotional, structural violence that happens when you're an outsider in a specific context and when it comes to something like fatphobia, it's much less inescapable. There's something about anti-fatness that adapts to every kind of environment. It's really hard to understand on how many levels I was failed because I was in the wrong body.

For Mikey, the intersections of race and gender also exposed them to a level of adultification that was confusing and left a mark on their memories of education in a P-12 setting. "I was adultified from a very young age, because my body was very different from that of my peers." Adultification bias happens to many youth of color, specifically to girls, where they are expected to "know better" and be caretakers, and may often be sexualized by adults around them.

> It was assumed that because I was bigger, I was supposed to be able to hold those kinds of expectations – how I related to my peers and the kinds of conversations I was

privy to or responsibilities that were placed on me [at home and at school].

Oppressive systems further project sexism, anti-fatness, and racism onto students of color in fat bodies. For girls, their physical development happening more quickly makes them susceptible to inappropriate and frequently sexualized treatment (and being blamed for drawing that attention to themselves). "When I think of my K-12 experiences," Mikey said,

> I think of being watched in ways I should not have been watched. And when I was a kid I would wonder if I was doing something to expose myself to that kind of attention. I think I felt really drawn to the idea of being wanted by people when so much of my life was defined by not being wanted because of my body.

Mikey shared an anecdote of such treatment from her teachers in a memory, she said, she thinks about it "almost every day."

> When I was in eighth grade, I was sitting in an English class next to another student who I had known since like, kindergarten – but we'd gone in two different directions at this point. He leaned over and pulled the strap of my bra down and my teacher got so much more angry at me than at him. She gasped and had this really intense, red face and sent him out of the room, but kept me after class to tell me "that was extremely inappropriate." I was being punished for basically being interacted with [without my consent] in a sexual way. The reaction was also completely outsized to the ones other students got [for similar behavior]. That one has stuck with me for so long, even though it's not the only one of that kind that I have, because it was a Black teacher, and I was surrounded by students I had grown up with, everything was so familiar – but in that moment I felt like a complete stranger. It was my first time truly feeling alienated from everyone around me.

The rules punish fat Black and Latinx girls more harshly – sometimes, simply for existing. Dress codes with "fingertip length" rules, such as the one I had in my middle school, which was strictly enforced, and high school, applied disproportionately to girls with larger bodies than thin ones. Mikey's experiences echoed my own in this way: "It always felt like a punishment for existing in space as a fat young girl." A study about adultification bias in youth of color from Georgetown Law confirms Mikey's experience. It found that "Black girls as young as five years old were perceived as being less needing of protection and nurturing, compared to their white counterparts."[38]

Anti-fatness is just another way that school systems can, have and do marginalize, criminalize, and push out (fat) Black girls through disproportionately enforced, fatphobic dress codes, anti-fat cultural bias, and arbitrary and disparate disciplinary measures. And as this study reveals, the narratives we continue to tell them in school about their families, their bodies, and their Blackness have led us to believe that they are "less bothered" by it. I don't buy that. Paul Campos notes that "fat hatred can often serve as a mask for other, often unconscious, forms of prejudice that manifest themselves when observers feel no compunction about expressing the fear and loathing that the sight of fat elicits in them." He also finds that several studies, including one from the University of Arizona, suggest that Black and Hispanic girls "tend to have much more positive body images than white girls."[34] This notion that Black girls are "less bothered" by weight-based bullying is inherently racist. We are supposed to believe that their tolerance of others' individual and systemic bigotry is synonymous with natural resilience; what's really happening is that in a system that does not value fat Black girls, and as a result they are socially conditioned to accept and internalize the social stigmas that form the nexus between anti-fatness, anti-Blackness, and sexism. Obesity researchers have found over the past two decades that girls of color have a lower rate of eating disorders, and also weigh more. Even still, diet industry titans like Jenny Craig and Weight Watchers have targeted much of their advertising toward middle-class women of color, likewise with kid-facing health programs like Let's Move! and

FitnessGram.[34] White women and girls often associate fatness with disgust and disdain, with the help of those same weight loss companies – who offer them the key to having a better, that is, *thinner*, body. Thinness has become a cultural extension of socially constructed power dynamics, and intersects and overlaps with race in ways that play out in the classroom, cafeteria, and on the playground. If "cultural competency" and "diversity, equity and inclusion," are co-opted in these formats, it has the potential to insinuate that the bodies of girls of color are in need of "fixing," because they are too confident in themselves and need help to maintain "reasonable" weight and size – of course, for their health. With this in play, companies that sell weight loss can only maintain a successful business model if they "make Black and Hispanic girls as neurotic about their weight as white girls tend to be."

For Black boys in fat bodies, it creates a heightened sense of stereotype threat. Adultification bias is a cousin of anti-fatness, anti-Blackness, and other forms of oppression that justifies violence against specific bodies. Largeness is more threatening, and Black boys in fat bodies are more likely to be seen as men or as if they are more "dangerous." It happens in the form of criminal justice systems, seeing them as men who should be held accountable through carceral systems like detention, suspension, and even prison – not as boys who, like any adolescent, have the ability to make decisions and mistakes that they can learn from. They often aren't given the chance.

Such bias was used to justify the death of Mike Brown, an 18-year-old teenager who was shot in the back in Ferguson, Missouri, after being suspected of stealing from a local corner store in 2014. Officer Darren Wilson, who shot him in the back and killed him, compared him to "Hulk Hogan" and a "demon." It is notable that Wilson also stated, in the full context of that quote, "I felt like a five-year-old holding onto Hulk Hogan," despite the fact that Brown was unarmed and Wilson was equipped with both a taser and his service weapon.[39]

Shortly after Mike Brown's murder followed the death of Tamir Rice, a 12-year-old shot to death in Cleveland for playing in a park with a toy gun. After his death, he was described by the The Cleveland Police Patrolmen's Association president said "Tamir Rice is in the wrong. He's menacing. He's 5-feet-7, 191 pounds. He wasn't that little kid you're seeing in pictures. He's a 12-year-old in an adult body."[39] The officer who killed him, Timothy Loehmann, arrived on the scene and within a fraction of a second, fatally shot Tamir. The assessment that was made in this instance? Fat + Black + toy gun = dangerous. From this statement, it appears that in the eyes of the state (including the prosecutor who echoed the adultification bias mentioned above), the highest crime Tamir committed was being fat, Black, and a kid with a toy in a public space.

Both these instances highlight not only the issue of the manufactured "threat" posed to the public, to law enforcement, and society at large by the existence of Black boys and men in larger bodies; it juxtaposes it with a presumed universal white innocence and virtue, especially in the case of justifying physical, psychological, and even fatal violence.

In the crosswalk where adultification, racism, classism, and violence meet, anti-fat bias is not often part of the conversation; but it needs to be. Many acknowledge the blatant fatphobia leveled at victims of police brutality like Eric Garner, whose fat body was blamed for not being able to tolerate the chokehold that killed him on a sidewalk in New York City. His last words, "I can't breathe," were used for racist, fatphobic jokes and Facebook discourse about why he "had it coming."

But the problem of blaming children – fat, Black children – specifically for their deaths because of the fact of their fat, Black bodies – has yet to be a significant part of mainstream social justice discourse. Violence against Black bodies is normalized, despite our supposed "awakening" as a nation after the murder of George Floyd; but we still rationalize the deaths of and body and spirit that Black, fat bodies are subject to everyday because fatness does not grant one proximity to virtue, to goodness, to inherent worth.

> **Quick Tip**
>
> For more about the intersections between race, violence, school, fatness, and adultification, I recommend two texts: Heavy: An American Memoir by Kiese Laymon and Pushout: The Criminalization of Black Girls in Schools by Monique W. Morris.

Being thin will not save us; but being fat guarantees that the world believes that violence is deserved or even expected – especially for fat, Black bodies.

No Thank You, Next

School-sanctioned weight labeling and teaching students nutrition using BMI and terms like "overweight" and "obese" as a framework for their understanding of bodies and identity go against the very ethos of the anti-bullying laws that remain on record as active policy in 49 of the 50 United States. If we know the history of anti-fatness and its issues in our social, economic, and educational fabric, that is the only way we will, as educators and school professionals, be able to do something different. If we do what we've always done, we'll get what we've always gotten: more social and systemic harm and inequity that hurts our kids. Also, the stereotypical bully we all see in movies and media almost often *is* a fat kid – but what are we doing to examine the ways that hurt kids go on to hurt other kids? We do not examine enough how the systems that legislate away bullying also, however unintentionally, create the conditions for it.

Besides the flawed, racist, cissexist, and ableist history of BMI and its lack of usefulness in telling us anything about the "health" of students inside our schools, it begs the question: what is being done with this data to address the disparities it claims to illuminate? Does knowing this information then prompt policymakers to provide stigma-free nutrition or assess so-called "food deserts" in their communities? In a 2020 Medium article, Mikey Mercedes argues that the idea of "food deserts" "can obscure the fact that these are not naturally occurring features of the environment, but something inflicted by some groups of people on others."[(40)] And the obsession with "food deserts" may be compounding the fatphobia levied at the people who live within them. Mercedes states:

> The other major reason why the public health field loves talking about "food deserts"…is its general disdain for fat people. "Food deserts" have long been connected to

rates of "obesity," a long time fixation of public health>
For those who are invested in "obesity prevention," the
issue of "food deserts" is another way to link fatness to
badness and moralize food. "Food deserts" witht heir
typical overrepresenattion of "ultraprocessed" foods and
underrepresentation of fresh "healthy" foods, are bad
because they have too much bad food and not enough
good food. In turn, people in "food deserts" are fat and,
as most in public health would say, fat is bad. Therefore
"food deserts" are bad because they make people fat.[40]

In uncoupling fatness and lack of morality or willpower, we must
interrogate not just the systems that built these associations, but
the systems that blame fat people for their very bodies. What
is our society doing to mitigate the social factors that lead to
poor health (independent of weight) for those communities – is
it lowering their cost of living? Is it paving a pathway to more
affordable and accessible health care for their families? Without
solutions, framing this data as a "problem" stemming from the
"obesity epidemic" only deepens stigma experienced by fat, poor
people of color, and frames fatness, not social inequality and
systemic oppression, as the problem. Lessons and framing that
paints a picture of food deserts as moral battlegrounds where the
people living in them deserve pity, instead of equity, access, and
care, are not telling the entire story.

Many studies reflect that obesity is an indicator of poor
performance in school, or that fatness is correlated with low
grades; but what appears to be missing is that actually, weight
stigma is often what's causing poor grades. The narrative about
fat students has long been that they are lazy, less capable, and
teachers are not exempt from displaying this bias. Though it has
been studied most heavily in physical education teachers, which
makes sense, because much of their work has to do with fitness
and the entanglement of movement, perceptions of fat bias,
physical activity, and health indicators, teachers across subjects
and grades display size bias and weight stigma in not only their
attitudes and treatment of students, but maybe even their grading
practices. Literature on teachers' grading in school "posits that

grades are not always a fair measure of subject-specific competencies because they can also reflect teachers' attitudes about the students."[41] Unfair grading practices because of these attitudes, namely weight stigma, can and do impact students' willingness to learn, show up to school, and their overall wellbeing. In their study of students' grade outcomes in German and mathematics (the study was done on students in Germany), Mona Dian and Moris Triventi found that among German seventh graders, "the incidence of children who received a low grade is largest among obese students, decreases but stays rather high among overweight students and is lower among normal weight students."[41]

Research published in the *British Journal of Educational Psychology* in 2019 indicated that middle and high school English teachers also grade according to tropes about students in larger bodies. In the study, teachers assessed the quality of a contrived student essay assignment, accompanied by photographs of the "student" who was supposed to have written each essay. The researchers asked teachers to provide perceptions of student effort, overall success in school, and the need for remediation and tutoring, as well as a grade for their work. They also asked teachers to reflect on their thoughts about their own grading biases and those of other educators. The essays supposedly written by students who were "overweight" were "judged to be similar in structural quality,"[42] but were assigned lower grades compared to "normal" weight peers. The 133 teachers surveyed also reported that they assumed students who were "overweight" needed more tutoring, had lower grades, and probably had to try harder to complete the assignment. They also suggested that other teachers were probably more biased when grading students based on attitudes toward specific students, but didn't think they had the same level of bias themselves.[42]

I know that when faced with all the ways that weight stigma inevitably does harm in a school system, the outlook can feel bleak. In the next few chapters, we'll investigate, interrogate, and aim to address the problem, piece by piece. Along the way, we'll go through the various places, spaces, and situations where anti-fat bias might arise at school; and some "fat equity fixes" you can tangibly use to make schools more equitable for the students you teach, and even the colleagues you work alongside every day. The rest of this book calls on all of us to teach students to trust their bodies so that they can bring their full, true, and whole selves to a learning space. The tasks our bodies perform to keep us alive every day are nothing short of a marvel – and teaching students from the perspective of body trust, safety, and acceptance are paramount to making our classrooms places where students can, and want to, keep learning.

RUN IT BACK: Reflecting on Your Practice

♦ *How does anti-fat bias intersect with other oppressive ideas and structures such as racism, sexism, adultification, ableism, transphobia, and queerphobia?*
♦ *Where is anti-fat bias present in your school?*
♦ *Does your school have any policy that addresses weight stigma or anti-fat bias explicitly? What does it say?*

3

"We've Been Waiting for You"
Changing the Built Environment

Good teaching and meaningful learning can happen anywhere. School as we know it is a space, a physical place that houses not only learning, but belonging. Before students can learn and teachers can teach, we have to set up the space for teaching and learning and belonging.

But how can we do this before knowing who our students are? There's so much to consider: How will we arrange the furniture? How much space does our room have? What kind of furniture do we need, and what do we already have available?

Too often, we ask these questions *after* students have entered our rooms. It's hard as rosters change, as kids grow, and as engagement waxes and wanes and we rearrange the room on a whim just to "change it up." But one thing that should not waver is what the space we design tells the students we teach: that how they show up is welcome and it matters.

Dr. Bilal Polson, an elementary school assistant principal on Long Island, started his career as a physical education teacher; he has a keen sense of what it means to be flexible and build sustainably inclusive learning environments.

DOI: 10.4324/9781003534143-4

Giving teachers environmental autonomy is critical, and making sure the messaging is clear that this is not a bank or a factory, it's a learning environment. That means that different students need different things at different times of day.

In his school, Dr. Polson says the classrooms have "scoopy chairs," students can work and write and draw on the floor, sit in a traditional or standing desk, and many classrooms have futons or tables. In his own office, he sits on a stool to ensure he is attentive to the task at hand. This modeling ensures that there is no "standard" way to sit or learn, and that flexibility and diversity of needs are honored in student learning processes and outcomes. This is especially critical for students in larger bodies, because finding them seating that helps them feel secure often means they stand out.

If the desk arrangements, or even the desks themselves, do not tell students that their bodies belong, that they fit – we cannot expect them to learn safely and comfortably. Attached desks or chairs with arms often send this message to students with fat bodies; suggesting that if you don't fit here, you don't fit *in* here. In their essay for *The Fat Studies Reader* (2009), Ashley Hetrick and Derek Attig state:

> [Attached] desks, are not, we argue, neutral and benign spaces…[they] seek to both indoctrinate students' bodies and minds into the middle class values of restraint and discipline, and inscribe the messages onto the bodies that sit in them…at the heart of desk design is the issue of containment, the protection of rigid spatial boundaries and uncompromising values that, paradoxically, both highlight and erase the bodies that refuse to conform.[43]

We cannot expect students to learn only once and only if their bodies comply. And, especially for students with disabilities and access needs; we cannot wait until they arrive to shift the space that they occupy for a significant time each day. Our room should not treat students' bodies, mobility aids, or needs as an afterthought, but a part of the classroom environment. We cannot wait until a chair breaks or an attached desk pinches their skin. If we modify our classroom after they arrive, they learn that it's not important to have these accommodations ready in anticipation of diverse needs and differences. But if we have adjustable furniture, if the desks are unattached and armless, and rows aren't tight – students can hear and see, instead, "we've been waiting for you."

If you must seat students in rows, make sure they have enough room to pass through the rows without squeezing or bumping into someone else. For fat kids, says Crystal Maldonado, YA author of the book *Fat Chance Charlie Vega*, "it's a flashing arrow pointing at your differences." Things like rows and attached desks, and too-small bleachers are "physical reminders" of the differences fat students face – because what goes through their minds is often, "Can this chair support my weight? I don't want to inconvenience anyone with my body." She says,

> Fat kids have so much more to worry about than their peers, and it's built into their environment. Like, how is this space going to possibly, literally reject my body and make me feel mortified? If you break a chair, that is going to stay with you for the rest of your life.

Oftentimes, the people who design these spaces overlook this issue until something like that happens – and the student who it happens to is often the subject of bullying, taunting, and humiliation ever after. What if our classroom geography, from the minute the students walked into the room, says health teacher Kerri Tracy, tells students "we've been waiting for you," instead of "we'll figure it out after you get here?" The former approach signals to students that we were thinking about them and what they might need before they even landed on our class roster; the latter suggests their needs are an afterthought, and to them, may feel like a burden. We can't afford to wait until a chair breaks or a desk is too small. Creating spaces that welcome all isn't a flexible seating fad; it's a necessity.

It's not just desks in the classroom that pose an accessibility problem; it's the chairs with arms in the counseling office, the auditorium seats that squish students together too closely, and cafeteria benches that ensnare the legs under the table and make a spectacle of leaving your seat. The latter especially is a form of messaging: don't leave your seat; it disrupts order. When we do not, as a system, invest in students' comfort and ease, it makes it harder for them to learn anything other than how to conform.

Big Moves for Classroom Setup

◆ *Chairs without arms – in the classroom, in the library, in the auditorium*
◆ *Normalize "alternative" seating that anyone can use, anytime (beanbags, cushions, benches)*
◆ *Desks and chairs that separate*
◆ *Sturdy seats*
◆ *Walkable perimeters around tables*
◆ *Just say no to rows*

Anti-Fat Bias and Curriculum Violence

Just like anti-fat bias permeates our individual and collective consciousness often whether or not we know it, it also permeates our curriculum. Curriculum violence has often been taught through the lens of race and racial trauma, but anti-fat bias being taught as a cautionary tale is also a form of curriculum violence. According to Learning For Justice, "Two Black scholars, Erhabor Ighodaro and Greg Wiggan, coined the term curriculum violence in their 2010 work *Curriculum Violence: America's New Civil Rights Issue*. They defined it as a 'deliberate manipulation of academic programming' which 'compromises the intellectual or psychological well-being of learners'."[44] The ways that trauma happens to fat students in the context of their P-12 school experience doesn't have to involve being ridiculed, shoved into lockers, called names or humiliated in the cafeteria to constitute as violence. It doesn't even have to be intentional to be detrimental, Jones argues.

When we envision the curriculum violence experienced by fat students at school, people's minds typically sprint straight toward health and physical education. But, from my experience, fatphobia is ubiquitous across our content areas, across grade levels, and potentially present in any classroom – not just the gym. It can come in the form of misunderstanding correlation and causation in math, leaning on outdated or bad data in science, not studying the history of dehumanization of fat people in social studies, and a lack of equanimous representation of fat bodies, and the people who live in them, in literature. As an English teacher, I'm often asked why (besides it being personal) anti-fat bias matters so much – and even told it's not "my lane" as an educator, because I teach reading, writing, and literature – not health. But the potential for harm and trauma happens across grade levels, across subject areas, through what we teach; just as much as what we leave out or what biases are inherited and passed down to students from their teachers. Constant refraining that "fat is bad" codifies anti-fat bias leads to internalized anti-fat bias in fat students and internalized dominance in thin ones, creating the conditions for harm to be done outside the classroom. Though often associated with doctors, teachers invested in equity of all kinds must follow the rule of "first, do no harm" in their classrooms, including in the subject areas they teach.

In the following sections, we will break down common ways that curriculum violence takes shape across grade levels and content areas, and how teachers can strive to plan, think, and teach differently to minimize the harm that curriculum does to our students, irrespective of their size.

Just a (Fat) Kid, and Life Is a Nightmare

Early childhood education is a golden opportunity to teach kids lessons that will stay with them for life. With this opportunity comes the opportunity to teach children about size diversity, joyful movement, and that being in a body is an inherently good thing.

Several studies done in the past few decades suggest that between the ages of three and five, children start internalizing messages about their bodies, about size, and come to value the thin ideal.[45, 46] Longitudinal studies have also found that this awareness and internalization of the belief that "thin is good" increases with age.[47] This means that teachers, parents, and adults in a child's life can shape how they see others, see themselves, and see the world – for better or for worse.

For their real-life peers, weight bias in preschool-age children means that kids assign negative attributes, such as lazy, mean, ugly, less intelligent, and sad to people in larger bodies, and positive attributes such as friendly, successful, and intelligent to thin ones. They are also less likely to choose a larger-bodied peer to be their friend in social situations.[48, 49]

Most studies tracing anti-fat bias in preschool-age children, however, study two-dimensional representations of fat bodies such as line drawings, attributing adjectives such as "strong" to drawings of thin people and "stupid" to drawings of fat people. In their 2013 findings, John Worobey and Harriet Worobey found that "Since much of preschool-age children's knowledge is gained via their interacting with concrete objects, the use of dolls could serve as more tangible if not necessary realistic stimuli for assessing attitudes toward body shapes."[50] They created their own "doll test" to do just such an assessment among 3 ½ to 5 ½ year old girls.

In their doll test, the use of three-dimensional figures such as dolls was, at the time, a (surprisingly) unique method of studying weight bias in young children, particularly girls. Eighty-five percent of the 40 girls in the study owned at least one Barbie doll, and were asked to evaluate characteristics of each Barbie doll presented to them; a "thin" doll, an "average" sized doll, and a "fat" doll.

The girls were asked, among the three dolls – who had different-sized bodies, but the exact same head, and all were dressed alike – to identify which of the dolls they thought was smart, happy, pretty, assumed to put toys away, have a best friend, help others. They were also asked which doll they thought was likely to be sad, tired, have no friends, be teased, or eat the most. The results indicated that "the fat doll was least often selected on all six positive attributes, ranging from 47 percent for "no friends" to 67 percent for looking "tired."" The study also found that when asked the question of which doll they would prefer to play with, "70 percent of the girls chose the thin doll, followed by 20 percent choosing the average doll and 10 percent choosing the fat doll."[8] Researchers were especially struck by "the attribution of "pretty" to the thin doll by nearly two-thirds of the girls," despite them having identical heads and being dressed in the same outfits.

Researchers also found that toddlers and preschool-age children perceive fat characters as having negative traits like being "mean" or as villainous in their movies, books, and media.[51] that The study that Tutt references in her article is from 1998; where two researchers

> told preschool-age children two stories that portrayed one girl as "mean" and the other as "nice," and then asked them to indicate which figure was the mean or nice one. Averaged comparisons showed that the "chubby" figure was chosen as the mean one more frequently.[9, 50]

Another study from 2019 states that "Along with well-supported evolutionary theories of weight bias, including disease avoidance, innate disgust, and evolutionary fitness, a growing literature indicates that weight bias is learned or strengthened socially."[52] This harkens back to the ideas that Ancel Keys purported in his "seven countries" study; that health and disease are correlated, but not causal; but that in his opinion, being personally affronted and disgusted by fat bodies is enough to warrant doing something about it.

Marx et al. also state that

> One frequent source of stereotyping and biased portrayals is children's media programming...Despite often using magical or supernatural elements in a whimsical manner, children's media has historically promoted gender, race, age and weight-based stereotypes. Characters who are overweight are subject to ridicule, are less socially involved, and have fewer romantic relationships than their normal weight peers.[52]

This strongly supports the visible impact of cultivation theory – the idea that repeated and prolonged exposure to biased portrayals of a group or person perpetuates biased beliefs. If the makers of media carry that inherent bias, they have the power to perpetuate these biases in children's media to audiences that are impressionable and likely to internalize the idea that fatness makes one inferior, and then transmit that onto others. All of these studies make one thing clear: addressing weight stigma and anti-fat bias should begin as early as possible.

These portrayals are one example of the implicit messaging that fat = bad that happens before children even enter their formal school years; so that when they arrive, they come with a built-in understanding that being fat means being other, an outsider. In early childhood learning experiences such as read-alouds, teachers can reverse this narrative by choosing representations of fat bodies just existing, being joyous, being kind, being accepted, and feeling like a part of something.

My own first foray into this thinking was the character of Ursula in Disney's *The Little Mermaid*. She was an unapologetically fat sea witch who knew what she wanted – a voice. She is portrayed as evil, manipulative, and ultimately, the villain. In fact, this paradigm is mentioned in the Marx research study, which sought to compare weight bias among preschool-aged children toward both non-human cartoons and human figures. They reviewed the previously mentioned studies of line drawings and dolls, and concluded that "children hold biases against overweight figures regardless of the level of stimulus realism" – meaning that a character can be drawn, three-dimensional, or human – the weight bias still holds firm. They also cite researchers who found that in early elementary age (ages six to eight), young children express stronger thin-ideal attitudes following exposure to programming with animated thin characters. Marx et al.'s study utilized both human, alien, and non-human characters with different body structures, depicting them as both "good" and "bad" in personality or behavior – and still found that the negative traits; the participants attributed traits like "mean," "lazy," "stupid," and "ugly" most frequently to larger bodied and alien characters; revealing that not only was a fat-bias schema intact in children in their study, but so was an aversion to the unfamiliar or "alien." They also found that anti-fat bias was more frequently leveled against girl figures by the participants in general. The schema for learned bias against outsiders, fat individuals, and gender bias meets here, and as these and other research have found, it is pervasive, begins early, and maintains throughout early childhood. Marx and his co-researchers conclude that "The more often unconventional heroes in media become the norm, the more opportunities children have to associate a variety of characteristics with being desirable, weakening weight bias."[52]

In alignment with their research of animated and non-human figures, Marx et al offer the main characters in the animated Pixar movie *Monsters, Inc.* as a counter narrative to weight bias in young children. In the film, the two main characters, Mike, a short, round, one-eyed green monster and Sully, a large, fluffy, fat monster are both the heroes of the story, while Randall, their antagonist, is the story's villain.[52] Representations such as this can offer children critical skills that enable them to see that traits such as "mean" aren't limited to a body type or gender. They also argue in their conclusion that the wider representation of bodies and personalities may "provide an avenue to intervene in prevention of weight-based bullying, allowing children with a variety of characteristics to identify with their heroes and stand up against weight bias."

*   *   *

Early childhood education settings are also huge opportunities to help kids build a positive relationship with food and movement. Schools structure most of a child's day without their input, and though this makes it easier on the adults in their lives and teaches them about concepts such as time and transition, it can also whittle away the intuitive eating and movement mechanisms that we are born with before the construct of scheduling, convenience, and the everyday hustle of life gets in the way. Physical therapist Mary Lynn Hafner asserts that "developmentally focused movement activities help children form active habits, discover their bodies, learn self-control, improve self-esteem, increase independence, and build self confidence."[53] She emphasizes guidance, support, and joy rather than competition in the early stages of children's development, stating that "If we have a secure foundation in learning movement strategies during our early years, these early experiences will overflow into other areas like language acquisition and social emotional development."[53]

Aisha Atkinson (she/her) is an Instructional Leader in Stafford, Texas whose district serves a community of learners six months to six years old. When we spoke about her experience as an educator and an administrator in the early childhood grade band, she noted the curriculum is "severely lacking" in representation of size. With scripted curriculums like Amplify, which make some effort at diversifying representation in the texts that they make available to students, Aisha noted that in fairytales, for example, characters are depicted as slim, described as "fair," and teachers will prompt students with questions like "what does this word mean?" and affirm answers that make these characteristics synonymous with beauty and being "pretty."

> The images being shown [to students] are not of people of varying sizes. We are instead continuing to perpetuate stereotypes of physical fitness looks like someone who is always in the gym, very slim or very toned. It does not look like a person who is plus-sized living their best life and making choices that best fit.

Aisha observes. She also noted the impact that mnemonic devices serve on the process of internalizing narrow representations of health, fitness, and beauty have on children in the early childhood education stage of their development.

> When it comes down to internalization for students when you are showing them an image, hearing it with music, and reinforcing it with actions and movement, you're developing multiple layers of memory and retention of information and knowledge within the child. And of course, that causes children to grow up with unhealthy images of what health actually looks like.

These memory devices, which are critical to student retention, thinking, and learning at an early age, may also carry with them an implicit curriculum that causes students to view things like health and wellness in binary terms.

Aisha gave the example of Jack Hartmann, who composes these kinds of songs for student learning, and whose Youtube channel opens with the tagline "Jack's music is research-based and teacher-approved to focus on helping children learn important state, national, and early childhood standards."[54] One of his songs, "Let's Get Fit" helps children count to one hundred by ones, and doing exercises or movement while counting. The opening lyric is "Count to one hundred every day / keep your mind and body in shape / let's get fit, have some fun / count to one hundred by ones." The song is set to a pop-rock beat and repeats the first verse again after counting to 100.

Movement, counting, and wellness are all acquired, important, lifelong skills, and songs like Hartmann's put all those skills into one place; but when coupled with images of only one specific body, one way of being – these songs can pave a path to implicit bias. In Chapter 3, we will further explore the corporate, government, and other ties that Alisha's home state has to fitness initiatives that may help stigma take shape.

Using music and movement to retain information is a really important balance to strike. I would be curious to see how teachers define "fit" for students, or whether fitness is standardized and synonymized with "thin." I also wonder, what is "in shape" in this context, and how is it defined? Words have an impact, and are used intentionally when forming schemas like the ones children associate with their bodies, their self-esteem, and self-image. Similarly, the word "fat" and its associations carry a stigma that begins early. In preschool and kindergarten, students develop an awareness that being fat is bad, and associate it with characteristics such as mean, lazy, stupid, and lonely. The earlier we frame it as a descriptor like tall, short, or thin, the less charged with negative connotation it can become, and the less frequently "fat" may be used as a pejorative term loaded with disgust to make their peers feel inferior.

I also spoke to Joana Mandoli (she/her), an early childhood educator in Oregon, about her experience helping students and families in a special education early childhood setting with maintaining this intuition while learning how to communicate their individual needs. She describes what she does as "pre-preschool," because it is a setting in which parents are present in a preschool setting to help their children adjust and learn skills like communication, socialization, and other structures that many neurodivergent kids need support around before entering school.

"In our preschool setting, everything is an invitation; you can go to snack, you can go outside, you can go to feeding time...but none of those things are demands that we put on kids," she said. We spoke about the importance of invitation, especially to things like movement and mealtimes. At the age of early childhood, convenience and time-management on part of the parents (and teachers/school systems) often trumps a child's intuitive, innate hunger, and fullness cues.

> **Quick Tip**
>
> If a child expresses they're hungry and it's not "time to eat," be flexible; ghrelin (our hunger hormone) doesn't wait until snack time!

One thing that we do in a preschool and kindergarten setting is that snack time is from this time to this time and there are no meals or snacks outside of those times. But what I know as a special educator is that meals are really challenging for a lot of kids.

Joana continued to think about her experiences with neurodivergent kids, food, and classroom structures.

What we know in special education is that the link between things like autism and eating disorders or obsessive compulsive disorder and eating disorders are pretty closely linked because it's a real space of control and power and knowing your body,

she said. Indeed, the link between "picky eaters" and neurodivergence and disability is strong – but forcing kids into the "clean plate club" and having them sit until their plates are finished just doesn't work. Instead, it creates an imbalance of power that is characteristic of compliance, control and sends a message to kids that the adults in the room know their bodies better than they do.

> A lot of the kids I work with are what we'd call extremely picky eaters or restrictive eaters. So giving parents permission and telling them it's okay for their kid to eat Ritz crackers all day and make mealtimes what's going to work for them helps kids feel a sense of control around food,

Joana said. As school becomes more and more structured, especially in early childhood where time is modulated into tasks and activities, a greater sense of agency and intuition over their eating lives is paramount. Even in places where diet variety is offered to children, trying new foods is a challenge that often becomes a battle and a power struggle between kids and adults – and they need to know that letting them stick to the foods they like isn't "taking the path of least resistance," it's a lesson in intuitive eating and body trust.

When Joana was a kindergarten teacher, she remembers a curriculum that introduced children to the idea of "go," "slow," and "whoa" foods. She said the messaging implied that "well, candy's not bad for you, but don't eat it!" and associated foods with stoplight colors to indicate what and how much was okay to eat. This kind of regulation mimics the same model as Kurbo, a food tracking app designed for children ages 11 and under by the weight loss company Weight Watchers (now rebranded to WW).

"[In her current classroom] We view meal time not as an eating opportunity but as a communication opportunity." In Joana's classroom, parents hold some of their kids' food and their kids are encouraged to find a way to request the food they want – whether it's by pointing, grunting, speaking, or gesturing. Anything they don't want to eat goes on a "no thank you plate" and is saved for later or not eaten, without judgment.

Giving children the ability to articulate that they're not hungry, that they don't want to eat (right now, or at all) is an important tool for fostering agency, regulation, and moving our educational institutions away from a culture of compliance and toward embodiment. Though Joana's role is to support neurodivergent children and their families, all students and families could benefit from a learning space that is free from judgment, expectation, frustration, and compliance-based monitoring (and the potential for developing hypervigilant self-monitoring) around food.

Intuitive eating and self-regulation also go hand in hand for children who are developing a sense of their hunger, fullness, likes, dislikes, and body image. "For instance," Joana said, "your kid might eat a bunch of candy and then they're not going to feel very good. We use something called "neutral commenting,"" which is commenting without assigning value. An example might be something like "Hey, you ate all your Halloween candy, and now you have a stomach ache; I wonder if those two things are connected," she said.

> I didn't assign value to the candy with a comment like the candy is going to make you fat or give you diabetes or rot out all your teeth, but I invited them to think about how food makes them feel.

An important aspect of the learning process in early childhood education is movement. As Aisha Atkinson highlighted earlier in this chapter, movement is an important part of learning, retaining, and integrating information into the developing brain; it helps produce schema and helps young children process information. But movement is all too often presented in school settings as a means of "fitness," and this has the potential to also create schemas in children that uphold diet culture.

Movement can instead be used to help kids begin to self-regulate, and as a tool for processing more than just learned pieces of concrete information; it can help with modulating feelings and thoughts, too – and as a way of bringing the body back to a baseline that feels comfortable and safe so that they can continue learning, growing and engaging in their environment.

"In the preschool setting where I am now, we discuss movement as a way to regulate ourselves; we don't need to attach value to it," Joana said. Helping students think about how they want to feel or what tasks they want to accomplish that day and what food they will need in order to do those things is a more helpful, intuitive way to think about food and movement, instead of using either as compensation, or in pursuit of the thin ideal or "fitness."

"We talk a lot about food and movement in the context of what it does for us, our bodies and our brains, which I think is a better approach," Joana said. "The question we want to be asking ourselves is, 'do you feel the way you want to feel?' and 'are you able to do what you want to do?'" she said. "If you asked me or my friends those questions as a kid in the early 2000s, the answer would have been "I want to feel skinny," and now, I know that's not really a feeling."

> **Quick Tip**
>
> Rethink "fat" as a feeling word. Try aiming for more precise language through investigation of your physical and emotional states: are you bloated? Feeling tired? Sluggish? Lacking energy? Once you get the hang of it, model this for those around you.

Joana talked about using "heavy work" as a movement philosophy, which involves moving heavy objects from one space to another. Her students help with moving and carrying chairs to gather for snack time, putting away toys, and setting up the classroom space to help students regulate and move their bodies. This resembles some parts of the cognitive behavioral therapy practice of TIPP, which stands for temperature, intense exercise, paced breathing, and progressive muscle relaxation; but adds on the idea of participating in community as a means of movement and regulation.

They use trampolines, slides, "puppy jugs" and encourage running. Instead of individualized "staying fit" attitudes toward movement, Joana's students can focus on regulatory activities that have more than one purpose; lifting heavy objects to help her students manage their emotions and get moving, taking turns using the slide or the trampoline. At home, she and her teachers encourage parents to have their kids help bring in groceries or carry laundry. These practices help encourage movement while participating in community and being involved in creating and sharing space together. "If it helps get them moving *and* they're being helpful, that's like a one-two punch in terms of toddler care."

Early childhood is perhaps the most important time to get started in creating equitable, stigma-free spaces for our children and their bodies. It is indeed an opportunity to teach them that their bodies, all bodies, are valuable, worthy, and important and that they can trust themselves to eat, move, be, and grow at their own pace.

Big Moves for Early Childhood Educators

◆ Be flexible about when kids eat; if they're hungry, create space to honor their hunger and support what their bodies are telling them.
◆ Encourage movement that is community-oriented, fun, and free from "fitness" rhetoric or diet culture.
◆ Leave behind the "clean plate club" expectation; start a "no thank you" plate and normalize revisiting or refusing food that students don't want to eat.
◆ Use movement and food as a communication opportunity and an opportunity for self-regulation.
◆ Seek curriculum resources with diverse representations of sizes and equally diverse portrayals of characters, people, and figures with different sizes.
◆ Ask students questions that encourage them to think critically about how bodies are represented, instead of prompts that reinforce weight bias schema.
◆ Have students make their own self-regulation or movement tools to encourage fine motor skills in addition to self-regulation; stress balls, calming jars, and "puppy jugs" (milk jugs filled with sand, with a puppy face drawn on and a leash attached that they can "take for a walk").

When the COVID-19 pandemic struck in 2020, students and teachers experienced a colossal shift to online learning. Students' homes became the classroom out of necessity and uncertainty at what the onset of coronavirus would bring.

As the pandemic wears on and COVID continues to persist, fat people and our bodies are, unsurprisingly, caught in the crossfire of conversations about health, personal responsibility, and access to care. Fat bodies themselves have been treated as an epidemic for decades; the response to fat people with COVID and the perception that fat people were bringing yet another plague upon ourselves for being fat – is tremendously prevalent.

In an article for Danish pop culture blog *Konfront*, Dina Amlund writes:

> Every time a fat person falls ill – whether it is a broken bone, having allergies, depression, asthma, anything at all – if the person is fat, their fatness will be blamed and weight loss will be proposed as a solution and there will be either explicit or implicit blame of this fat person being at fault and having caused it by being fat.[55]

In a study published in the *Journal of Pediatric Psychology*, Dr. Leah Lessard and Dr. Rebecca Puhl determined that "Despite an absence of empirical evidence, narrative commentaries have called attention to the upsurge in derogatory and blame-ladened portrayals of obesity during the COVID-19 pandemic (e.g., memes about gaining weight and overeating)."[56]

Aside from the added fear of being told by society that my weight was the cause for alarm, now society, and medical communities worldwide, suggested that my weight was a problem because it would make COVID more likely to contract and more difficult to overcome. And this was not making me feel less anxious about becoming ill with the virus, which I did twice in two years. The overlap of the "obesity epidemic," especially the childhood obesity epidemic, put still more stress and blame on the bodies of fat people for potentially becoming ill with COVID, and fat bodies were (and still are) made to be a "burden" on the healthcare system for needing respirators, ventilators, and hospitalization to overcome the virus. Women's studies researcher Karisa Butler-Wall puts it most succinctly: "As scapegoats for larger social anxieties over national fitness and changing patterns of production and consumption, fat bodies have emerged as a primary target of "a vast network of surveillance, monitoring and regulating strategies and technologies" by medical, government, and corporate agencies."[57] Later, we will discuss how these technologies, corporate influences, and the government work together to monitor the bodies of P-12 students through digital and curriculum tools such as the FitnessGram®, school lunch program contracts, and youth fitness.

Weight stigma also remained active in the consciousness of teens and adolescents during the early onset of the pandemic. Lessard and Puhl's survey of over 400 students ages 11–17 found that "on average, 45% of adolescents reported increases in seeing jokes on social media about people eating food because they are stressed, whereas 46% indicated no changes in stress eating jokes and only 9% noted a decrease."[56]

They also found that "Additionally, increases in seeing memes about people gaining weight on social media were reported by 37% of adolescents, while 51% reported no changes, and 12% indicated decreases in viewing weight gain memes."[56] Puhl's earlier research on social media and weight stigma finds that when internalized, jokes and memes such as this can impact the ways that young people see themselves and the bodies of others. The two researchers agree, concluding that

> While joking can function as an effective tool to positively reappraise stressful situations, it is important that individuals are encouraged to utilize strategies to cope with pandemic-related challenges and stress that do not imply personal responsibility and blame for body weight.[56]

The kinds of rhetoric that happened early on during the COVID-19 pandemic about bodies, BMI, comorbidity, and fatness scared and emotionally activated me as a fat adult, so I cannot imagine what kinds of fear it instilled into my students. I tried my best to focus on helping students maintain their mental health, sleep hygiene, and relationship to technology through a balance of activities they enjoyed. I went out on a lot of walks out of sheer boredom and a need to get out of the house and breathe fresh air, safely away from others.

Quick Tip

Help students become responsible consumers of content by learning to recognize weight-stigmatizing language and phrasing. Is it a joke that is meant to make someone else feel bad about their body?

The notion that fat bodies are a burden on society, inherently unhealthy, and an epidemic to be eliminated just for existing was underscored by the threat posed to *everyone* of all shapes and sizes by COVID-19. Amlund focuses on the ways that problematic rhetoric about fat people and our bodies leads to blaming our "obvious" lack of health for the prevalence of COVID among fat people, treating us like a disease to stay away from, now for more than just one "good" reason. COVID disabled many Americans, and many fat Americans – but substandard healthcare has been disabling fat Americans for a long time.

School was supposed to close for two weeks, then the closure lengthened again, until finally we were told to come retrieve our items from the building in shifts while masked, and stay apart. Brief check-ins via Google Meet slowly became longer, full-period classes as we realized we wouldn't be returning for the year.

The following year and the year after that, the norm of having at least half the class joining in from home on a screen was something I was used to. I would teach the students in the room, while carrying a laptop and teaching the other half of the class who was on Google Meet. There were disconnections, misconnections, and as much laughter and joy as we could muster in these weird times when relationship building was made harder by learning from home.

What I wasn't ready for was how much time I'd spend talking to myself when it came to virtual teaching; sometimes, it was difficult to know if students were even there on the other side of the screen. And sometimes, *they weren't*.

Teaching to students remotely had many people involved in the school community at-large asking questions about education and access: parents, teachers, administrators, counselors, and students alike. For some students, being able to learn from home was the first time that learning felt accessible, paced on their terms. For other students, it was a logistical nightmare, especially for reasons related to technology and internet reliability, childcare needs, scheduling, setting tech boundaries, and social-emotional wellbeing. For fat students in particular, learning from home meant that attached desks, locker rooms, and other places where fat bodies are often subject to humiliation for the sake of education were no longer a problem.

I was really distracted by the way my face looked on camera, and at the time, didn't know the "hide self view" option was even a thing in video calls. I can only imagine how students who experience body dysmorphia must have felt, especially within systems that required "cameras on" for attendance purposes to ensure students were present, attentive, and engaged during lessons. Lessard and Puhl's research echoed my questions in their findings:

> Adolescents' perceived changes in body dissatisfaction were aligned with changes in their exposure to and experiences of weight stigma during the pandemic. For example, adolescents reported increased body dissatisfaction of 64% and 63% after exposure to stress eating jokes and weight gain memes on social media, respectively.[56]

I thought a lot about how appearance-based bullying might be ramped up because of policies like "cameras on"; in an age where everything can be captured, screenshotted, shared, and distributed in seconds, how were schools protecting the privacy and dignity of students while ensuring they were accountable for attending class from home? This has yet to be confirmed by studies, but would make sense given the prevalence and presence of social media in the lives of teens, especially teens with not much else to do but scroll on a phone from home. "Within the peer context, while reduced time spent in school (e.g., via remote learning) may lessen the frequency of targeted peer weight-related mistreatment, it is possible that in person bullying has been replaced by electronic (cyber) bullying."[56]

Were there, are there, more creative ways to get students to engage without making them distracted by their appearance in such a visceral way?

The combination of doubled-down medical and media rhetoric about fatness, COVID, and comorbidity certainly has the potential to increase not only body dissatisfaction, but weight-related hypervigilance and self-monitoring; especially in adolescents, who display "heightened sensitivity to social input"[58] and "concern for appearance"[59] as it is.

This rise in unstructured time, combined with the enormous stress of the pandemic and its far-reaching consequences, has led to widespread concerns among the general public about vulnerability to overeating, sedentary behavior, and weight gain. These concerns are reflected in the explosion of social media posts referencing the "quarantine-15,"

notes Rebecca Pearl.[60] Everyone, especially teens, looked to social media during lockdown for entertainment and a way to stave off isolation boredom; but many also looked for support, encouragement, and safety – especially those whose home and family dynamics included a lack of support to begin with.

While many found support online for maintaining healthy habits (myself included), teens remain especially vulnerable to stigmatizing social media messaging and content for two reasons: (a) they know how to navigate it and utilize a wider range of applications more than most adults in their lives and (b) the adolescent brain is vulnerable to social input. Additionally, kids are often immersed in a culture that conflates the appearance of thinness with health. So for many people, including many young people, social media was, and is, a pandemic escape. Considering all these factors, the rise in input of weight-stigmatizing messaging may very well have created more fear and anxiety around body image.

Pearl states that

many of the recent coronavirus-related posts have included text and visual content that convey strong fears of gaining weight or becoming "fat." A quick search of "#quarantine15" yields more than 30,000 Instagram posts [as of my research in 2024, more than 59,000], not including thousands of posts using related phrases (e.g., "COVID-15") and those found on Twitter and Facebook.[61, 60]

She argues that

These types of portrayals elicit common stereotypes that people with obesity are lazy and slovenly, and that they lack self-control (1). They also imply that having a higher body weight is an intolerable problem to be avoided at all costs (quarantine-related messages that promote unrealistic thin ideals and extreme weight control practices have been flagged as dangerous by eating disorder advocates as well).[22]

Messaging like this produces more distress for people already vulnerable to food struggles, reinforcing a "why bother?" mentality by making weight gain seem inevitable. Experimental evidence has shown that exposure to weight stigma actually increases high caloric intake and binging behavior, especially among people who are already fat, due to a rise in cortisol and stress response. Being repeatedly told you're going to die from your body's size, and then told you will die from your body's size *and* from a deadly virus, isn't exactly easy on the adrenal glands.

The thing is, even if COVID-related weight gain were universal and ubiquitous: the experience of anti-fat oppression is not. For people already in fat bodies before the onset of COVID-19, various systems already blamed us for the ways we existed; blamed us for being a "burden," and would continue this stigma by blaming our bodies for becoming sick with a virus that did not, that does not, pick and choose who acquires it. Our bodies are not inherently disabling: the systems that refuse to care for them equitably are.

Four years later, all those photos of folks who gained weight at home have turned into weight loss promotions for getting rid of their "pandemic weight," marketing campaigns for products that the diet industry has been peddling for decades, and quippy jokes about "needing to social distance from the kitchen, because I tested positive for a big ass."[57] How do we expect kids and teens to maintain their mental health if the prevailing message is that weight is another thing on their list to have anxiety about *during a global public health crisis*?

Big Moves for Remote or Virtual Teaching

◆ State upfront that cameras are optional, and create other ways for students to check in. Be explicit about why and for whom that option is created; it will help those who benefit from it most feel seen.

◆ Check in with students in the chat; find alternative ways to assess their attendance throughout a class session (emoji react, breakout rooms, attendance questions, whiteboard responses).

◆ Establish virtual classroom agreements with students, including the sharing of peoples' information, likeness, or voices; make respect for privacy and a shame-free environment an expectation of all who participate in the learning space.

RUN IT BACK – Reflecting on Your Practice

◆ *How has the pandemic impacted my own body image in relation to my role as an educator?*

◆ *What power and influence do I have to begin conversations about weight stigma as early in the year, or as early in my students' educational journeys, as possible?*

◆ *What associations and narratives are my students building about bodies and body size? How can I help?*

4

The Health/Phys Ed Trauma Is Over (If You Want It)

Health, PE, and Anti-Fat Bias

Rethinking Health(y)

Our obsession with weight has fostered, especially in the United States and the global "west," a set of "societal norms and values that continue to prize thinness and allow (and even encourage fat shaming, where fat individuals are scrutinized constantly and judged for their health related choices"[3] Thin has become synonymous with "healthy," and "fitness" has become a proxy for weight loss.

As a matter of fact, various studies done across the 1980s and 1990s have found that being over average weight is a protective factor for longevity, including a watershed longitudinal study done in Norway that followed 1.8 million people for ten years. Despite the American medical establishment's claim that a BMI of 18.5–24.9 is "normal" or "optimal" the study found that the highest life expectancy of 79.7 years was found among

DOI: 10.4324/9781003534143-5

people with a BMI of 26–28. People who were underweight according to the BMI (18–20 percent body fat) had a lower life expectancy than those with BMI percentages between 34 and 36.[34] More studies (Ernsberger, Haskew & Andres, International Collaborative Group, First National Health and Nutrition Examination Survey) found similar results, affirming the idea expressed by Paul Campos in his book *The Obesity Myth* that "in almost all large-scale epidemiological studies little or no correlation between weight and health for a large majority of the population – and indeed what correlation exists suggests that it is more dangerous to be just a few pounds 'underweight' than dozens of pounds 'overweight'."[34]

As such, given the ubiquity of such values and attitudes in our society, the curriculum in schools has reflected this cultural and social value.

> While many people can get behind the idea that cellulite is normal, and that we don't all need to look like Kate Moss or one of the Kardashians, there is still a common perception that self-acceptance is only allowed up to a certain size, at which point shrinking our kids' body is not about beauty – it's about health.[4]

Much of the conversation about body positivity, body size acceptance, and dismantling anti-fatness begins with "but what about health?" and from a pedagogical perspective, I'm going to do my best to answer that question for teachers.

Fear, Loathing and Food Diaries

A popular figure used to create fear and anxiety around fatness is this number: 300,000. The prediction which became a popular health assertion was based on "a previous study that tracked fewer than two hundred actual deaths out of the 115,000 (excluding smokers) women it surveyed."[19] The study excluded smoking from the data, even though smoking and nicotine have widely been used as a way to stay thin; especially among women.[19]

This number, a supposed death sentence claiming that "three hundred thousand people in the United States die from obesity per year" has been cited in the media thousands of times. For such a massive number and an earth-shattering claim, the sample used to defend it was rather small, showing methodological issues. The *Journal of the American Medical Association* agreed; and in 1998, in a statement which read that the figure was "by no means well established…derived from weak or incomplete data."[19] The study's data indicate that persons with a BMI of 20 run the same risk of premature death as those with BMIs of 30, even though the former are "ideally" thin, and the latter are "obese."[34]

Medical professionals and organizations repeated this enough times that it was used as the argument to approve weight loss drugs like Redux in 1996, and became the linchpin for FDA approval for future diet drugs that would enter the market.[19] Once again, fear of fat, not objective health science, won out, and this culture of fear has trickled down into our schools.

Like many teens and adolescents, I did not leave my health and physical education classes unscathed. While I was fortunate enough not to be in the class that watched *Supersize Me*, I had teachers who taught health who, as part of our "nutrition education" suggested that eating any single food item containing 200 or more calories was "unhealthy." No mention of the other contents – macro or micronutrients, sugar, etc. – just a caloric assessment of over 200 was enough to make a single food untouchable. I would apply this food rule later in my restrictive eating patterns, and it has stuck with me. It's hard not to cringe every time I read a food label and see a number larger than two in the hundredths place, even if it's an entire meal. In her article "Is Your Kid Learning Diet Culture at School?," Oona Miller Hanson states: "Students who change their eating habits according to school lessons can quickly become nervous around food, develop health anxiety, and get into caloric deficit that can catalyze an eating disorder."[62] I know that this was certainly true for me, starting in middle school and not ending until well past college.

What could have caused this is a lack of nutrition education for my teacher – leaving them to fill in the gaps with personal beliefs and patchwork information to guide their lessons. American students get, on average, eight to ten hours of nutrition education per school year.[63] Research data from 2013 indicates that only 11 percent of districts required nutrition education training or professional development for all staff, and only 8 percent required NE training for food service staff.[6] With a lack of consistency and oversight into sound, evidence-based nutrition guidelines and ongoing professional conversations about what that looks like when it becomes student-facing, we open up the Pandora's box of diet culture to enter conversations about health and wellness, as they did in my tenth-grade health class.

In 2022, a tweet I wrote in response to writer Molly Forbes' daughter being assigned a food diary at school in the UK went viral. My post simply read "Please stop assigning food diaries to students. Please."[64] I didn't expect it to garner much attention, but instantly and then overnight, it received almost 50,000 likes, over 300 replies, and 3,700 reposts. Parents reported that their kids received similar assignments and wouldn't be doing them; others reported that they were made to write food diaries in school, and it strengthened their disordered eating patterns or made them feel ashamed for their cultural foods, especially when teachers wrote comments about "too much" fats, carbs, or dairy. In the replies, I saw just how much food diaries, especially for an assignment, highlight and embarrass fat kids, poor kids, and reinforce negative weight control behaviors. When teachers comment on students' food choices using language and evaluative tools that are not value-free, and instead make judgments about what they eat, it positions students also to be and feel judged for who they *are*.

In 2004, filmmaker Morgan Spurlock released *Supersize Me*, a documentary-social experiment in which he went on to live exclusively off of fast food for thirty days. This film quickly became the norm to show in high school health classrooms, as "proof" that eating processed foods frequently enough would make you fat, fatigued, and miserable. At my high school, one teacher used it as a staple in their curriculum without fail every semester.

> This film is still shown to students as if it were simply a presentation of nutrition facts. Food documentaries—especially without any attention to media literacy and critical thinking—harm adolescents, who are already vulnerable to eating disorders and negative body image,

tweeted Oona Miller Hanson, educator, writer, and parent coach.[65] Websites like TeachersPayTeachers still have lesson plans, activities, and worksheets for teachers to use with the film to engage their students.

The same year Spurlock's film came out, then-U.S. Surgeon General Richard Carmona made notorious statements targeting obesity as "the terror within."[17, 66] Employing the same rhetoric of McCarthyism, Carmona asserted that the rise in obese children would affect military recruitment. He cited the (debunked) 300,000 statistic as his ammunition for the claim. This was especially potent rhetoric given that the country had faced the terrorist attacks of 9/11 two and a half years prior to painting a picture for all of America that the leading public health crisis and threat to our safety was not terrorism, but fatness. Once again, our nation's fitness levels were synonymous with national security.

As of this writing, *Supersize Me!* Creator Morgan Spurlock has passed away, at the age of 53 from complications related to cancer. News of his death revealed he also struggled with alcoholism for a lot of his life, including during the film's production.[67] The filmmakers conveniently left this detail out, even though it could have shed a more complete light on the alarming numbers related to his liver function after filming. Critics of the film say that it does not take into account the idea of socioeconomic disparity (which is a major reason for the boom of the convenience food industry in the first place) and frames food, and fatness, from a place of morality and privilege. Spurlock was able to access medical care and return to a stable diet of nutrient dense food. He presents his experiment by acknowledging it as something that people in America do regularly; but positions the ability to choose differently as if it is easy, accessible, or morally superior. Throughout the film, Spurlock meets several people who engage in the behaviors of fatness: one who eats two cheeseburgers a day, and has for years, but also jogs and does physical activity regularly. The man is in relatively good health. These examples parsed throughout the film are supposed to be a "gotcha," a cautionary tale, and highlight the supposed absurdity of an "obesity paradox." – the idea that fat or very fat people can somehow still be healthy "despite" their weight.[2, 66]

> These documentaries are a lot more engaging than a textbook chapter or a worksheet. And they might seem like a good replacement for food journals or other "healthy eating" assignments. The films are well-produced and very compelling. And that's exactly why these documentaries can be so dangerous,

says Oona Miller Hanson in a 2024 article for her Substack.[68] "Teens are deeply engaged in the process of exploring and forming their identity; suddenly adopting a new food identity can have serious health consequences."[68] Films like *Supersize Me!*, *Food, Inc.*, etc. are "crafted to entertain and persuade," and sometimes, they persuade adolescent viewers right into an anxious relationship with food. "You cannot unsee gruesome images of slaughterhouses or scary charts about mortality and disease (never mind that many of their conclusions are exaggerated or based on cherry-picked data)."[68]

It's Psychosocial – Understanding the Social Determinants of Health

Economist Robert Crawford coined the term *healthism* in 1980: the idea that our health is a personal responsibility, not social inequality or environment, and that in turn, fixing our lack of health was our responsibility, too.[2, 4] Healthism, in short, is rugged individualism of the body. In a highly individual society like the United States, individual responsibility as freedom (personal and national) has, unsurprisingly, given rise to the same principles applied to children's overall educational and curricular experiences.

In order to reframe and help students understand health, we first need to show them that health is so much more than an appearance, a performance, or a number on a scale. Health is about equity and justice. The social determinants of health, which include educational access and quality, access to quality healthcare, a safe neighborhood and built environment, social and community connections, and economic security illustrate this.[69] Christyna Johnson, RDN, adds things like safe drinking water, literacy, and nutrition access to the list.[70] While the CDC acknowledges that inequalities exist, they also still fund, perpetuate and engage in research and data that affirms the use of unreliable and unscientific measures like the BMI. In societies like the United States, economic disparity, lack of healthcare insurance coverage, and neighborhood conditions such as clean air and water, safe housing, and social support are lacking – and this needs to be part of the conversations our students have in health class. If we are going to expect them to move their bodies, treat their bodies well, and love their bodies, they need a more rigorous understanding of health rather than just an overview and some broad-brush science. This starts with inviting students to see the social conditions around them and connect these social conditions to the way their bodies move, feel, and live. The way health is taught to students must emphasize that it's not just a personal journey, it's also a collective effort.

Quick Tip

I first learned about "blue zones" from a fellow teacher at a PD. They are places in the world where longevity is attributed to physical activity, low stress, rich social interaction, low disease incidence and local, whole food consumption. Blue zones are, essentially, places where all the social determinants of health are accessible. They are considered the healthiest places on earth. Though their scientific efficacy remains to be seen through extensive research, they might offer us something to learn and teach about the social determinants of health and the importance of community in determining a healthy life.[71]

According to her article for SLATE, Natalia Mehlman Petrzela asserts that "PE is often on the budgetary chopping block and devalued even within the education profession as less important than academic subjects."[72] Only a handful of states make physical education a requirement, and an even smaller number of schools host physical education classes daily. What's equally important to maintaining the integrity of robust programming for physical education in schools, however, is how we implement it. If we are not intentional about the ways we teach health and physical education, which includes students' relationship to food and movement, we cannot progress toward a curriculum that prioritizes their true wellbeing. Instead, we make them live in fear of disease, acting out of a sense of anxiety and shame rather than embodiment, community, and self-care.

In this way, school health curriculum has become more about constructing the *appearance* of health through long-accepted myths and political agendas rather than about evidence and objectivity.[73] Policies, people, and private interests have moved the goalposts for what health education entails since before we conflated weight with health in the past century and a half. Researcher Aubrey Gordon found that "Weight wasn't thought of as a primary indicator of health until the late 19th century, when life insurance companies created charts of ideal weights in order to figure out how and what to charge policyholders".[2] The tables reflected only those who could afford life insurance, and were created by mathematicians and sales reps, but not any actual medical professionals. Like the early BMI, measures were fixated on an "ideal," but this time they were pushing a product.

Environments also have the power to enable health-promoting behaviors, and Bauer et al argue that "school physical and social environments may be especially important influences on the dietary and physical activity patterns" of students, especially in early adolescence.[74] ""Getting healthy" is aspirational, optimistic, laudable. It seems to eschewed size, instead prioritizing health, but quietly, implicitly links the two...For years, "getting healthy" has paved the way for conflating fatness with ill health," says Aubrey Gordon, in her book "You Just Need to Lose Weight" *and 19 Other Myths We Tell Fat People.*[2] This kind of mindset around health, especially when it turns into school curriculum, asks students to perform what they think is healthy, and often that means, what they believe will lead to thinness.

> **Quick Tip**
>
> *Encourage students to be hyperlocal in their approach to health: what accessibility do they have to health-promoting behaviors, a healthy built environment, and other social determinants of health? What or who does not have access? Interrogate the space around you as you define and develop a definition of health in your classroom.*

In their book *Body Respect* – the same one that colleagues laughed me out of the faculty room for reading at my first teaching gig – Lindo Bacon and Lucy Aphramor unpack many myths about children's health. Beginning with the fear mongering that America's kids are getting fatter, they cite the National Health and Nutrition Examination Survey, which indicates that actually, American kids' weights have been relatively stable since 1999, and that there is no data supporting the common media assertion that today's kids will have shorter lives than those of their parents.[75]

Calories in, Calories Out Is OUT

"It's just a matter of calories in, calories out; it's not that difficult." Sound familiar?

For a discussion about producing and using energy, this equation is rather simple. But our bodies are not simple machines like the kinds we learned about in physics class, and only *kind of, sometimes,* fully adhere to the above statement which captures the law of conservation of energy we learn in science. Our bodies are much more complex, and what our food is made of is even more complex than that.

The guidelines taught in health class about nutrition rarely cover this complexity and the nuances of food, nutrition, and health. This oversimplified and oft-repeated understanding of the ways our bodies work to process energy gives calories a bad reputation.

Calories, especially in "excess," are thought to lead to fatness – and fatness has the worst societal reputation of all. One origin for this bad rap is the 1959 paper by Max Wishnofsky,[2] who claimed that each pound lost or gained "had a caloric equivalent" of 3,500 calories. This figure came from his analysis of existing literature on weight loss, and has since been disproven. As we've learned with most of what we think we know about nutrition, the key isn't reliability of evidence, but reliability of repetition of supposed evidence. Not all calories are created equal;[76] calories from fat, for example, may be absorbed differently than carbohydrates.

The social determinants of health *must* be part of the conversation we are having in class about nutrition; especially considering that not all bodies use calories the same way. Several factors contribute to the ways energy is used, absorbed, and/or stored in the human body: genetics (over a hundred of them affect food absorption), disease, gut bacteria, medications, stress responses, and even the entry of plastics and other chemicals into the blood which change our body's metabolic and hormonal processes over time.[75] So, two differently sized people can eat the same breakfast, lunch and dinner, and due to the perfect storm of factors leading up to the absorption of that food into their bodies, have different outcomes on the scale after eating. If nothing else, this emphasizes the need to look more closely at the ways that access to care, clean and green spaces, and social inequalities play a role in health. If we oversimplify the ways that nutrition works for our students, we are effectively hiding the whole truth from them about health. Teaching health with this level of specificity would require more health classes, not less. And if we're going to undo weight stigma, it starts with students having a more comprehensive understanding of how their bodies work. Equity begs us to move beyond glossing over the trendy or novel topics; if they're important, current, and happening now, we ought to spend time on them.

Mental Health = Health

Trends in health education dictate the focus of health classes, from drunk driving education to drug prevention to mental health. Since the pandemic, there has been a push to include mental health education in health classes. Behind car accidents, suicide is the leading cause of death among adolescents.[77] More than just a trend, mental health education can offer valuable tools for students to engage in self-regulation, compassion, and even identifying the signs of crisis in themselves and their peers. It's important that mental health education be seen as not a standalone topic, but part of their overall health. What if we integrated mental health education to include the rest of the body?

Stress management is typically attached to the teaching of mental health in schools. The connection between health and stress is an important one, and stress even has the power to "turn on" or "turn off" certain gene expressions in our bodies.[75] The body's physiological response to stress, or allostatic load, is a contributing factor to disease in the body. Helping students see these connections through health and science paves the road to teaching skills like executive functioning, distress tolerance, time-management, and opens up conversations as a school system about how to reduce that load on our kids. Again, it bears repeating that in many cases, school is a stressor for students. Teaching them how to manage stress is a moot point when we are creating stressful, high-pressure academic environments that do not address inequity, or that uphold diet culture through tacit reinforcement of the thin ideal.

Body image issues among school-aged children have been at an all-time high, especially among secondary students. The average onset age for restrictive dieting is age nine among girls in the United States.[9] Our nation's inconsistent messaging about food – when, where, what, and how much to eat – is not only confusing for students, but irresponsible. To combat these mixed messages, educators can work together to help students individualize their choices, teach complete and accurate information about food, health, and movement, and discuss the in-depth consequences of restrictive dieting and eating disorders. Liz Browne (she/her), a social worker at an urban middle school, notes that girls are wearing bigger, baggier clothes. A reason she cites for this fashion shift among the students she works with is the increased volume of students that is common in the transition from elementary to middle school means more classmates to compare themselves to. Among the boys, she says, the motivation to engage in movement to get stronger, she says, also has motivations in performing and defining masculinity by a narrow set of cultural standards. She says that despite the specialized focus on social-emotional learning at her school, name calling and bullying having to do with body image is often coded behind other microaggressions – she talked about conversations with students about how calling someone a "fat bitch" is both fatphobic and misogynistic; and reports that in her experience, bullying among boys that is body-focused is often tied to implied teasing about sexuality and manliness.

Another thing Liz reflected on is the potential for mind-body connections during health class on students' executive functioning and mood regulation.

> Being encouraged to listen to their body and understand why they're feeling something – sometimes, hunger can look like aggression. Giving them the tools to connect the dots between hungry, angry and upset would be explosive for students, in a good way.

She noted that she felt like students in middle and high school would be especially open to this shift in conversation and feel empowered by it, especially as they grow and engage in activities like sports.

Liz, who has been at her school for six years and remembers, like I do, how weight control was a staple of our middle school experience, says that though students are "less afraid to eat" than we were in class or in the cafeteria and less likely to skip meals. But helping students understand that *what* they eat and *when* they eat, she says, warrants further discussion. "This year was the first year our cafeteria offered a salad bar, and so many kids didn't know what that was or how to combine foods to create a meal they'd enjoy," she said. "[Our school] will lecture them about health and [now] give them access to salad, but make other food that isn't appealing and doesn't look edible." She also told me about a poster outside the nurse's office that she said felt strategically placed; it read "Burn calories, not energy!"

The irony of posters like this is that by definition, calories *are* energy. Demonizing calories opens up the door to disordered eating behavior and a fraught lifelong relationship with food and movement (I know from experience). The anti-calorie crusade, once again, is mostly directly linked to our universal fear of becoming fat and a misapplication of all the other factors that determine our individual body's caloric absorption. According to Dr. Renee Anushka Alli, "a healthy amount of calories depends on a person's age, height, and activity level. It can change from day to day, especially if they are still growing."[78] Well into high school, many students' bodies are still growing, and as they participate in team sports and other activities that demand more energy from them, it becomes ever more important for students to see calories as their friend and understand how *their* bodies work to use them. Teens and young adults remain the highest risk group for eating disorders. Among reasons for developing these disorders, researchers cite fear of weight gain, guilt, and shame around food, thinking about dieting, and a desire to be thin as predictive factors for eating disorder development in young adults.[79] Restrictive dieting and even laxative and diet pill abuse are especially important to talk to adolescents about in the context of health, because adequate nutrition helps their bodies grow; and disrupting this process can impact them in the short and long term.

The average age of development for eating disorders among adolescents in America is 12–13 years old.[80] Often when we think of eating disorders, the imagination fills in for us a picture of an emaciated person, and typically female. Despite media representation to the contrary, eating disorders do not have a body type, can affect all genders, and are increasing in prevalence among school-age children. Anorexia nervosa can manifest itself as restrictive eating behaviors meant to control a person's weight, shape, or size and lead to malnutrition and malabsorption of nutrients, regardless of whether the person with the illness is clinically underweight. This is often called "atypical anorexia," but the only thing that's "atypical" about it is our assumption that thinness qualifies someone to have an eating disorder worth intervening in.[81] Anorexia is also the most fatal eating disorder, and the most fatal mental illness in general.[80]

Eating disorders among boys are garnering attention as well. Consistent with what Liz Browne said earlier in this chapter, the focus for boys and body image is one that often links directly with their notions of masculinity and performing the "ideal man." Besides the prevalence of anorexia, bulimia and binge eating disorder among boys, health professionals have noted the presence of muscular dysmorphia, colloquially known as "bigorexia," or compulsive eating and exercise behaviors shaped and motivated by the desire to gain muscle and lose fat.[82] The National Eating Disorders Association (NEDA) cites research from 2015 that indicates that 50 percent of preadolescent boys and 30 percent of preadolescent girls dislike their bodies.[83] A study from the University of Minnesota found that students who have access to how food works to fuel their body are less likely to develop depression, body dissatisfaction, adult onset binge eating behaviors, and attempts at extreme weight control.[78] Thinking back to chapter two when I spoke to Joana Mandoli, we can discuss calories in the context of "eating how you want to feel," and eating so that your body can do what you'd like it to. This includes thinking, studying, and focusing on academic tasks, which most people don't think about when they think about energy consumption and usage. And a reminder we may need to help students with: "skinny" is not a feeling.

Brain Stew

Teaching and learning is structured, generally, in the form of units of study that are done in isolation. What if, like the way our bodies work, our learning about health and wellness was integrated, too? We cannot teach or view nutrition intake, for example, in isolation. As demonstrated broadly in the social determinants of health, our lives and our health are the result of a number of factors: behavior, psycho-social interactions, genes, economic security, policies, and our environment.[75] What we put into our bodies (as a result of food availability, affordability, and choice) is just as critical as what and who our bodies are surrounded by (a combination of systems, structures, access, and choice) – all of which affects our brains. It's why we emphasize to students that getting enough sleep and eating a good breakfast are important for functioning well at school; but that's just the beginning. In an interview for *The Puberty Podcast*, health educator Christopher Pepper said about high school health:

> I find it's really empowering to teach kids about how their brains are developing. I think of it as a strengths-based approach. You're saying "This is a time in life where this really cool thing is happening, while your brain is changing in a dramatic way — you're building the brain that you're going to have for the rest of your life. It's a time in life where you can learn things really fast. It's also a time where your brain is particularly vulnerable to anything that you expose it to." If somebody is taking drugs or drinking when their brain is developing, it can have a bigger effect than it might have on someone who's at a different stage in their life.[84]

He also said during the interview that his job as a health educator involves teaching communication skills and sustainable habits; but frustration arises when he has to "spend [time] combating misinformation that people have learned from friends, from family members, or have picked up online."[84] He emphasizes that reducing misinformation that students encounter is connected to their understanding of health.

Ghrelin and Leptin

Ghrelin and leptin are our body's "hunger hormones," and they act in opposition to each other to tell us when to start and stop eating. These hormones are tied to our body's metabolism, and a malfunction in their production can disrupt our body's natural ability to send us hunger and fullness cues.[85] Along with other hormones like insulin, which regulates blood sugar and helps reduce ghrelin after we eat (effectively shutting off our hunger signals once we are full), and cortisol, the stress hormone that stimulates ghrelin, signaling our bodies to consume energy so we can escape danger in the event of stress. Other hormones that work with these heavy hitters are peptides, found in our stomach to aid in digestion, and our reproductive hormones.[86] Changes in these hormones happen rapidly during puberty, which can explain why teenagers seem to "eat their parents out of house and home."

Quick Tip

Instead of food diaries, introduce students to hunger and fullness cues (many nutritionists develop them as tools for clients!). Invite them to mindfully and thoughtfully consider their hunger and fullness cues over the course of a period of time. Follow up with questions about energy levels, caloric needs, and sleep patterns to illustrate that hunger, fullness, and energy aren't universal.

Puberty and adolescence are a crucial time not to disrupt these normal hormonal processes. Teens' natural inclination to self-consciousness and identity formation butts up against their body's natural adjustment into physiological young adulthood. Especially for teen girls, eating in front of others is a source of anxiety, because they don't want to be seen as "stuffing their face"[74] even for having regular, normal eating behaviors. While their bodies are growing and changing at lightspeed, teens are more vulnerable to the language of food fear and fatphobia than ever. At this time in their lives, it's important to help students build resilience to their media consumption of the thin ideal while helping them understand the importance of engaging in balanced, health-promoting behaviors: maintaining a regular eating schedule (skipping meals can lead to ghrelin spikes and stimulate binge behavior), limiting processed foods and opting for more nutrient density (without the shaming language of "junk" food layered over it), adequate sleep hygiene, regular movement, and hydration. As we'll discuss further in chapter six, the alarming increase in kids dieting, juxtaposed with the decrease in age of onset of restrictive dieting behaviors, is actually worse for their ghrelin and leptin – and can kickstart the weight gain they were trying to avoid because of anti-fat panic.

Many processed foods also contain endocrine disruptors like PFAS,[87] which are especially important to eat mindfully during puberty. This, however, does not mean that they have to be completely afraid of them – being simultaneously empowered to know what's in their food, how it affects their body, and how they want to feel, without encouraging them to feel fear or see the usual suspects, calories, and sugar, as the enemy. Chemicals like PFAs are not in the food itself, but the packaging and preparation methods – things like nonstick cookware, makeup, lotions, paint, pizza boxes, popcorn bags, and rain coats contain PFAs. Though processed foods continue to be demonized by diet culture, teaching students that they don't have to be *totally* eliminated is important for helping them balance the dopamine-chasing, perfectly okay desire to share a bag of Takis with their friends at lunch or opt for milk and cookies after a long, difficult test at school. Food as a social and self-regulating tool is a function of our mental health, too.

Serotonin

Mainstream knowledge of serotonin has increased in recent years, thanks in part to mental health de-stigmatization efforts on social media and beyond. However, the understanding of the neurotransmitter is often oversimplified as the "happy chemical" that occurs in our brains. First and foremost, it is a neurotransmitter, which, in short, means that it carries messages from the brain to other parts of the body to aid in the body's function; including digestion, wound healing, and even bone health. Students may be commercially familiar with its counterpart, *melatonin*, which is actually made of serotonin and helps regulate our body's fall asleep/wake up cues.[88]

Approximately ninety percent of the serotonin made in our body is in our gut, and the other ten percent lives in our brain; so what we eat can affect our motivation, mood, sleep, and memory.[88]

Teaching students about nutrition and brain science from a self-regulation and self-care perspective, rather than focusing on reduction and dieting, may be a good way to help them integrate their self-concept and internalize the importance of the alignment between physical and mental health. The production of this neurotransmitter is why carbohydrates are so important; they help keep everything running smoothly.

> **Big Moves for Health/PE Teachers**
>
> ◆ Mental health is health: encourage your department to include lessons that teach students about the social determinants of health, eating disorder prevention, stress management, and how to improve their executive functioning.
> ◆ Be intentional about your language around healthy behaviors, healthy foods, and size.
> ◆ If your district isn't already, be transparent about letting families know that they can opt their student out of BMI data collection.
> ◆ STOP assigning food diaries, especially for a grade.
> ◆ Stick to evidence-based nutrition lessons; don't impose personal food rules on students.

An Invitation to Keep Going

Health teacher Drew Miller (he/him) says that "health classes can be a transformative, fun, engaging experience," beyond worksheets, multiple choice quizzes, and "sports movies that are supposed to be inspiring." "Health class, he says, is so important because the content can be applied to change students' lives immediately."

For this reason precisely, we need *more* health from our classes, not less. Health teachers: If you're thinking "But I don't teach science, this stuff is too complicated!" The science of health is vast, daunting, and complex, yes; but no one's asking us to name every cell and know every function. Health and science are typically siloed in terms of content area, certification, and curriculum, but go hand-in-hand in helping students understand their bodies. Health happens in the body – and understanding the body beyond "calories in, calories out" is necessary for teaching about the body. During my conversation with Drew, he mentioned that in his case, nutrition education was framed as calories in/out, which we now know is an oversimplification of nutrition; and we cannot afford to oversimplify for our students, especially if it's because we are nervous about our own grasp of the content. Nutrition education aimed at teachers needs to be followed up with methods for teaching it, beyond generalizations and food log activities.

"The thing that was missing was joy," Drew said. Now, as a teacher, he aims to close these understanding gaps by talking about the social determinants of health, Health at Every Size, intuitive eating, and media literacy. "I hope for more discussions, articles and video content that isn't outdated cautionary movies," he said. "Health is also about ensuring I'm not promoting disordered eating."

One activity Drew and I spoke about was one he designs where he has students learn to spot fad diets using a set of criteria: red flags such as elimination, especially of essential nutrients; counting calories or nutrients; the promise of a "magic" food; and the premise of trusting products more than trusting the human body and what it was designed to do (detoxes, etc.). He expressed reservations that such activities might provide an instructional manual for dieting, and concern that these kinds of diets might encourage students to follow them. I challenge teachers to think about the framing in response to understandable fears like this one. Giving students space to be critical of diet culture and providing them with logical evidence of what to look out for and why it's harmful might actually be a protective factor against dieting and disordered eating behavior.

Consider this an invitation to collaborate with a biology teacher near you! It can feel massive to take on content that feels like it's "out of your lane," but take it from someone who's been told to "stay in her lane" regarding this very subject: the work of knowing the facts so we can facilitate spaces for kids to question, unlearn, and critically think about weight stigma is *everyone's* lane. We've worked really hard together to see the problem of anti-fat bias; teaching is one way we can stop the fire from spreading among our students, or at least, put out small fires when and where we are able. Knowing the basic roles of the compounds that our bodies use to maintain a relationship between our physical and mental health is the key to integrating students' understanding of their bodies in meaningful ways, which leads to lasting change in how they see and treat themselves, and how they see and treat one another.

Educators and administrators must create environments that are appropriately challenging, but not overwhelming, and certainly, ones that consistently uphold policies and curriculum that address the stress of weight stigma on students in larger bodies. Developing explicit policy that addresses body shaming, weight bias, and language around protecting the inherent dignity must also not be at odds with our practices and messaging about body size, body image, food consumption, and socialization around size diversity. Physical education is a place where all of these ideas meet, and historically, it has lacked inclusivity on a large scale for a number of reasons.

Get Fit or Die Trying (But Hopefully Not?)

The relationship between fitness and American schooling is a concept that traces back to the mid-20th century. As "white flight" took root around the Progressive era, city funds went to building more and more playgrounds in working-class neighborhoods, and "the physical education profession gained a strong foothold in public schools, focusing squarely on improving children's health and character through play and sport." The Great Depression eliminated many of these programs formally, but the desire to maintain a healthy and strong America remained intact. WPA programs were tailored to free outdoor recreation with the New Deal, and the Civilian Conservation Corps (CCC) recruited young men by promising them hard work as a way to build muscle (Figure 4.1).

Following WWII, America underwent the widespread threat of the Cold War. In 1945, the Office of Physical Fitness and the New York State War Council published several books, both titled *New York State Physical Fitness Standards – Evaluative Procedures in Physical Activities for Girls and Young Women* and *New York State Physical Fitness Standards – Evaluative Procedures*

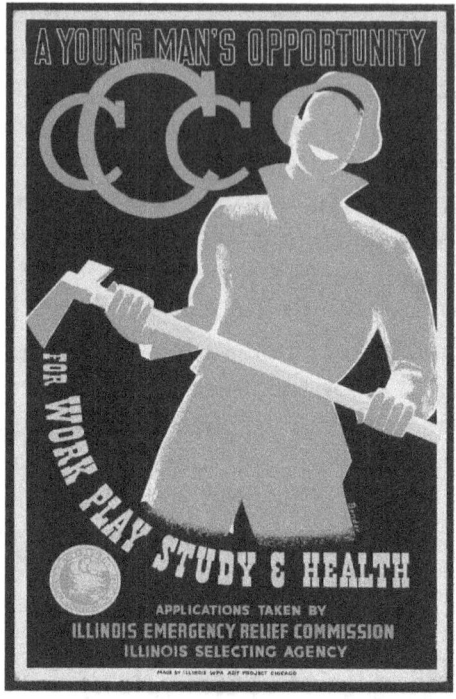

FIGURE 4.1 A Civilian Conservation Corps poster, WPA Illinois Art Project, Chicago, IL – Library of Congress.

in Physical Activities for Boys and Young Men.[89] As the tensions drew on, President Eisenhower feared Americans were not fit enough to fight if the war became hot. He came upon the research of two world-renowned mountain climbers, Hans Kraus and Bonnie Prudden, who later would advise him on what would become his President's Council on Youth Fitness in 1956.

Dr. Kraus, along with colleague Sonja Weber who worked with him at New York Presbyterian Hospital, developed the Kraus-Weber test;[90] a series of physical activities that tested a person's fitness level and took just ninety seconds to administer. The test consisted of a standard sit-up with knees bent and feet planted, a sit-up with legs extended, heel raises while lying on the back, trunk lift (raising head, chest, and shoulders off the floor while lying on the stomach), and bending forward to touch the floor with knees straight (later known as the "sit and reach").[89]

Its goal was to "strengthen the core, develop arm strength, and improve flexibility."[91]

They administered the test in 1955 to 3,000 children in countries like Switzerland, Austria, and Italy, with only an eight percent failure rate. Kraus and Weber remarked in their results that American children "have no bodies" and should "develop their muscles" through hallmark childhood activities like climbing more trees.[92, 93] Their vision of fitness did not, as later iterations did, seem to take the joy and fun out of movement; they just aimed to encourage more of it in America's children. On the surface, that's a great goal; move more, develop your body, and do things that build your esteem, character, and sense of adventure while doing it.

Enter Bonnie Prudden, a New York-based fitness enthusiast who administered and advocated for the use of the Kraus-Weber test and other fitness regimens, administered the test and other such exercise regimens on local children out of a converted school in Harrison, New York, which she bought and named the Institute for Physical Fitness. Inside the facility, chin-up bars were built into every doorway, and every child used the 42 stairs between the basement and top floor for "conditioning, discipline and special muscle building."[93, 94] At her Institute, she held exercise classes that began with her daughter's friends and then began studying the effects of the Kraus-Weber tests on local children. She found that 56.6 percent of school-age children out of a sample of 4,000, "failed." This finding became known as "the report that shocked the president" – and evolved into a government effort to pilot national fitness tests in school-aged children.

What ensued was an effort to strengthen kids through fitness tests that more closely resembled military exercises, endorsed and developed by the White House.[22, 23] In her subsequent writings, Prudden strengthens the link between fitness, personal responsibility, morality, diet culture marketing, and even national security. In her own words, she describes the results of her findings as "a terrible hullabaloo."[95] She says

The President said he was shocked and felt something had to be done, but most people started looking around for something that could take the blame. Was it the parents?

Was it the schools? What was it? The only thing they didn't blame was Communism. I've often wondered how they missed that; it would have been so convenient. As a matter of fact, if world Communists wanted to destroy us, they couldn't do better than we have been doing ourselves.[95]

Prudden asserted that America's physical education system has failed and stressed that fitness education in the "very aggressive countries of China and Russia" has not. The Sports Illustrated article that first introduced the data to the public consciousness called the findings "[a problem] which goes far deeper and has more serious implications for the future of the nation than many of those which haunt the news headlines daily."[91] This was the first time people's fitness level (and size) was being cast as a problem even more grave than national security. Even with nuclear war looming and racism and sexism in America booming, Americans' *bodies* were seen as the pressing issue of our nation.

Essentially, what became of this "fitness scare" was a response to the arms race – a sort of fitness race that would keep our country safe if we could just get kids to be more flexible and muscular. Prudden's statistics helped fossilize programming in physical education programs around the country.

What doesn't seem to be accounted for in her research is that the children she worked with had just survived a world war, and before that, the most pervasive economic depression in our nation's history. Food wasn't exactly abundant, and convenience food was growing in prevalence for mothers making meals while fathers were at war or at work. For the better part of a decade, America was in survival mode; and the bodies of American children adjusted to that accordingly.[72]

During her career as a self-made fitness guru (with proximity to privilege), she published several books, including *Bonnie Prudden's After Fifty Fitness Guide, How to Keep Your Child Fit from Birth to Six*, and *Teenage Fitness*. In the description of *How to Keep Your Child Fit* found on the official online store, it says:

Exercise for Babies? Isn't that carrying fitness a bit too far? Not according to Bonnie Prudden. Tests show that

American children don't meet minimum fitness standards and lag far behind European children in physical ability. Why? Lack of exercise in the first few years of life.[96]

In the description of *Teenage Fitness*, it reads:

A great body can be yours…go for it! You already know how important exercise is for your good looks, good feelings, and good performance – in school and out.[96]

Notice that the first thing that constitutes a "great body," according to this description, is looks.

The book description continues: *"So where do you start? That's easy. With Bonnie Prudden and Teenage Fitness. She'll guide you right from the beginning with the appropriate exercise for your needs – and you'll even have fun while you're building those muscles or firming those thighs!"*[96]

Quick Tip

Model different types of movement or modifications that all students can enjoy; ask your school to help creatively modify activities for all bodies so they can participate without stigma. Movement can benefit all classes, as students typically spend about three-quarters of their day seated at a desk. Incorporating movement into your lessons is a great way to get students to learn, think, and self-regulate; and a chance to help them see that exercise isn't all about changing the size and shape of our bodies.

Prudden described ways to keep children fit and offers her thoughts on the separate roles of mothers, fathers, and the nuclear family in maintaining not only fitness, but moral character (in her opinion, the two seem synonymous) – sandwiched between chapters like "The Backyard Track Meet" and "Swimming" is "A Union For Parents," which chides parents about "convenience foods" and the dangers of raising entitled children. The book parses advice about keeping kids fit using activities like running, swimming, horseback riding, dance, tennis, skiing, figure skating, and sending them to summer camp – all things that require equipment, clothing, coaching, transportation, time, and, of course, money.[97]

Fitness, like national security and moral character, was turned into an individual problem, and children were no exception. In *Teenage Fitness*, she speaks directly to her audience, telling them:

> When you came into school at the age of six, your parents had already softened, penned and pampered you to the point where 53.7 percent of you couldn't pass the minimum (Kraus-Weber) test; 43.6 percent were too weak, 32.2 percent were too inflexible. There may be some excuse for a man of eighty who has spent thirty years of his life under extreme pressure being tense and inflexible, but there certainly isn't for children of six.[95]

Though she published these kid-facing books in 1965 and 1972, respectively, it makes me wonder *which* American children Prudden is talking to and talking about – because for some American children, leaving their homes to play outside with their friends was due to lacking safe, clean, or green space, or even spaces free from racialized or other violence. It doesn't seem fair to blame kids, let alone their parents, for an America in which not only expensive classes, coaches, and equipment, but safe, clean neighborhoods are a privilege.

Yet, Prudden paints a picture of kids who were "kept in cribs, high chairs, toidy seats, baby carriages, car chairs, playpens, and strollers for much of their early years"[95] as a reason for their bodies' weakness and inflexibility. In this particular chapter, the blame falls simultaneously on the parents, and the children themselves. Prudden and the Council on Youth Fitness' response to the "softness" of American kids was tough love; they could either toughen up or let our nation fall apart. "In many ways, the perception that fatness is optional often allows prejudicial ideas and discriminatory actions to be couched as helping, encouraging."[3] Today's research suggests that shame-based comments about bodies, which are certainly not value-free, may actually increase weight stigma and drive people away from exercise and physical activity.[2] The conflation of weight with fitness and thinness "has developed societal norms and values (and spaces) where 'fat individuals are scrutinized constantly and judged for their health related choices.'"

Representations of what it means to be "fit" had (and still have) a certain body type, and Bonnie Prudden's work helped perpetuate still-pernicious thin ideals. It's no surprise that physical education teachers often display biased and negative attitudes toward fat people and students.[98] They are also more likely to assume that students in larger bodies cannot perform certain tasks because they are unfit, lazy, or less athletic; and that they were more impulsive, less organized, and had more family problems than non-obese people.[99] Such militancy around exercise hardly feels like a way to get kids moving in ways that are enjoyable. Left kids feeling ashamed, inadequate, and even further away from a life of liking movement.

Toughen Up for Victory

The year after developing the Council on Youth Fitness, a committee of federal officials – that included Bonnie Prudden and Dr. Hans Kraus – developed a pilot test that tasked Americans with completing pull-ups, sit-ups, the shuttle run (known by many coaches and athletes as "suicides"), the 50-yard dash, the softball throw (useful in softball games, of course, or for throwing a grenade in combat), and a 600-yard run. This remained the foundation of the fitness test for decades until the test was modified as a practice in the physical education curriculum in 2012.[92]

At one school in Carmichael, California, Coach Stan LePerotti adapted physical fitness exercises that measured students along fitness charts for activities such as timed sit-ups, push-ups, pull-ups, Prone backbends, finger extension push-ups, grip swings, bar hangs, and peg board climbing. Boys who participated competed for different colored trunks, which signified their achievements in these challenges.[100] Boys who earned "blue" trunks were required to best Navy plebes in pull-ups.

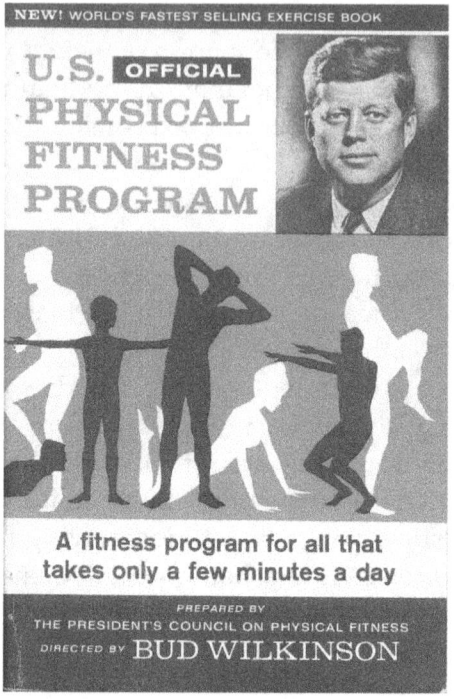

FIGURE 4.2 The official guide for the U.S. Presidential Fitness Program, compiled by
football coach and political figure Bud Wilkinson, who also contributed to
the program a theme song many know as "Chicken Fat."

This created an in-group/out-group culture of fitness among peers,
and served to motivate any "normal or even undeveloped boy" to
become a "superior physical type." In 1957 when these tests were
administered and developed, the Naval Academy qualifier for
pull-ups was two; at La Sierra, it was 13 (Figure 4.2).[101]

Inspired by La Sierra High School, John F. Kennedy famously expanded these policies and efforts. In a 1960 op-ed he
wrote for *Sports Illustrated* famously titled "The Soft American,"
he declared: "in a very real and immediate sense, our growing
softness, our increasing lack of physical fitness, is a menace to
our security."[102] This would be a first, but not the last, time that
the very bodies of Americans, and their lack of "vigah," would
be cast as a threat to the safety of our nation. JFK released a
booklet outlining his official fitness program, which was piloted
by nearly a quarter of a million students across six states.

For girls, participation in sports was unthinkable and seen as "unladylike."[72] The idea of "fitness" as a strategy for defeating foreign and domestic enemies remained under the thumb of the patriarchy. Though the standards resembled military training, the follow-through to enlisting and participating in military service was open only to men. So, while fitness was considered the American civic duty, adherence of "duty" to gender roles remained intact. Instead, fitness efforts aimed at women focused mostly on being able to perform the tasks of motherhood and on "reducing" (dieting). Equal access to sports was not federally guaranteed until the passage of the Educational Amendments Act in 1972, with the focus on gender and educational participation more widely known as Title IX.

*   *   *

While not being strongly linked to weight loss,[2] exercise is directly correlated with improvements in joint function, cardiovascular health, and mood.[3] The Cooper Institute for Aerobic Research, the creators and developers of the popular FitnessGram, cites that "Good aerobic capacity can reduce the risk of heart disease, stroke, and diabetes. Although generally not present in children, these diseases can begin during childhood and adolescence."[103] They also emphasize the importance of body composition in maintaining health. In their youth-facing materials available on their website, it states, "Overweight youth are at high risk for being overweight adults as well as having chronic adult conditions like prediabetes in childhood."[103] Thus, the maintenance of health is predicated on a fear that children might get these diseases because of fatness. The adultification of children's bodies is built into statements like these, which uphold and reinforce weight stigma. It goes on to say that "Adult obesity is associated with a number of chronic health problems as noted above. Since these health problems can begin early in life, it is important to begin healthy eating and regular activity early."[103] The assumption that fat kids become fat adults is a myth;[75] and, once again, centers "prevention" on fear and anxiety about disease that students may not, in reality, be genetically, environmentally, or behaviorally at risk for.

In the years since Eisenhower founded the PCYF, America has built and sustained a national physical education curriculum around shame; and cultivated in many Americans an aversion to movement. And what happened to fat kids wasn't inclusion in fitness initiatives – instead, they were met with an almost culturally sanctioned form of isolation, ostracism, and humiliation for what their bodies could not do. In an interview for *NPR*, physical education teacher Joanna Faerber said: "The test was totally backwards; We knew who was going to be last, and we were embarrassing them. We were pointing out their weakness."[104] It isn't just unrealistic to ask kids whose motor skills only just started developing to do a minimum number of pull-ups; it's cruel. "Rather than just giving me the dignity of letting me sit out or finding an alternative means of measuring my upper body strength," educator Aisha Atkinson said,

> I would be forced to go up, give it a try in front of my peers, knowing full well I couldn't do it – and be the butt of jokes for the rest of the day. Even in a society where we understand the importance of differentiation, we're still doing this.

It's not just their peers who are engaged in negativity and bias. In physical education classes, this can lead to students negatively evaluating themselves and their own bodies in a fitness context.[3] Students in all sized bodies need to see themselves in fitness contexts, and see themselves as capable models for movement just like their thin peers. In the realm of physical activity and education, language such as overweight "implies a proper weight to which all individuals must conform"[1] and ignores the realities of hormonal shifts, growth, and size, cultural and other forms of diversity that contribute to body composition in adolescents.

FitnessGram is touted as being "the most trusted and widely used fitness assessment, education and reporting tool in the world" (according to themselves) for gathering and analyzing data about student fitness levels. In 2012, after the Presidential

Fitness Test was phased out of the curriculum, FitnessGram was still widely used to assess as many as 22 million students in 2012.[105] In keeping with students' growing use in technology and social media, FitnessGram adapted into a digital tool that students use to self-monitor their progress in fitness, nutrition, and health through an online database. The intention behind this monitoring tool is to encourage students to "integrate healthy behaviors into their everyday lives, extending the field of physical education beyond the school walls."[106] On its face, this sounds like a sound goal, especially given the challenges students have faced with being more sedentary in the past four years due to COVID-related shutdowns.

FitnessGram bills itself as different from the Presidential Fitness test, because it shifts the focus from athletic performance on a fixed scale using fixed norms and competition with a percentile derived from the larger population.

> Fitnessgram is unique (and widely accepted) because the fitness assessments are evaluated using criterion-referenced standards. An advantage of criterion referenced standards (over percentile norms) is that they are based on how fit children and youth need to be for good health.[34]

According to their own website, FitnessGram results can be used to "track trends in fitness levels over time, examine relationships between fitness and academic performance and attendance, make physical education programs more effective, help create healthy school environments focused on prevention, and foster communication between teachers, parents, and students."[30] To their credit, the Cooper Institute cautions against "inappropriate uses" of the tool, and names using FitnessGram to grade students, using it as a sole criterion to "test students out" of PE, and evaluating the effectiveness of teachers as just some ways that the criterion and the software should not be used.[103]

In addition to being more precise, the ambition seems to also be to aim to help all students build positive attitudes toward fitness. There are no awards for achievement. The test consists of exercises such as a mile run, the Progressive Aerobic Cardiovascular Endurance Run (PACER) test, trunk lift, flexed arm hang, push-ups, modified pull-ups, and the sit and reach test, in which students place their feet onto a box with a measuring stick on top and must demonstrate the ability to flexibly reach forward. It also includes body fat percentage calculation and BMI calculation. The number of these tasks a student is able to complete, in addition to their body measurements, places them into a scientifically calculated Healthy Fitness Zone.

Steven Blair, the late renowned kinesiologist and once President and CEO of the Cooper Institute, once noted America's "misdirected and misguided obsession with weight and weight loss."[94] Similarly, the connection between weight loss, disease risk modulation, and exercise is increasingly intertwined, despite inconclusive and shoddy evidence that weight loss leads to significant changes in longevity; rather, fitness levels are a stronger indicator of long-term health, regardless of weight.[2, 34] In tying fitness levels to BMI as a scoring tool, FitnessGram seems to undercut its own value through the contradiction of equating fatness with a lack of fitness. Physical activity, regardless of a person's size, has various important health benefits, including but absolutely not limited to reducing disease risk, increasing mental health, lowering levels of stress, etc.[1] However, because we have culturally framed exercise and fitness as promises to deliver thinness, we create a culture around movement that is designed for people to give up. If it doesn't bring us to a smaller body, what's the point? America has one of the most sedentary cultures worldwide, and celebrating movement for the sake of movement is yet another contradiction that we ignore in the conversation about our health; if it doesn't bring us to the doorstep of the "perfect" (thin) body *right now*, we don't want it. And when we teach our students that fitness and movement are tied to pseudoscientific measures like the BMI and that every move they make that isn't tracked by an app doesn't "count," we muddle the messaging for them, too. Movement doesn't have to be about shrinking – and it's not empirically guaranteed to bring about much change in weight composition anyway.

The logic employed by FitnessGram appears more inclusive than JFK's visual of the "soft American": "While not everyone can be an elite athlete, most people can achieve healthy levels of fitness by performing the recommended amounts of physical activity."[103, 106] In guidance from Human Kinetics USA, it states that

> both fitness and fatness have stronger influences on health than previously suggested. The new standards reflect levels of fitness and fatness that provide protection against health risks associated with excess body fatness or inadequate fitness. The new standards have also resolved the previously mentioned problems with the previous standards.

The previous standards they're talking about were on a fixed binary – students either met satisfactory health requirements after doing the battery of tests or didn't. New standards label students as "passing" or "needs improvement" with a note after "NI" about varying risk of health conditions.[57, 106]

Through data and monitoring tools such as FitnessGram, students become part of a panoptic feedback loop: they are being tested, publicly and privately comparing themselves to their peers, and publicly and privately themselves to themselves. Could FitnessGram be another way for students to "discipline" themselves into the "right" body, especially if the framing is that physical activity helps them "control" and "regulate" their behavior?[57, 106] These data collection tools carry so much of the language of compliance, that it's hard not to imagine where and how it could go wrong; especially for students whose bodies are not privileged or socioculturally normative.

Emerging research has called into question the social-cultural ubiquitousness of this fitness test in international physical education curriculum. The FitnessGram privacy policy states they are FERPA-compliant, as well as compliant with educational privacy laws in the state of Texas (Chapter 38; Texas Education Code). The Texas Education Agency, a government municipality, forming a relationship with a company whose main source is student health data is just one example of the ways that bodies, school, and government are increasingly intertwined.

The FitnessGram itself, after all, is a product; and products exist to make people money. A striking number of Texas-based professionals are Cooper Institute trustees – including kinesiology professors, a tax lawyer, charity directors, several doctors, and even former Dallas Cowboys quarterback Troy Aikman. Creators of the FitnessGram also have ties to various publications, expensive research endeavors, and corporations in relation to academic publications, research careers, teacher professional organizations, critical scholarship (including some that promote healthism and weight stigma) and corporations like Campbell's Soup, the NFL, and SHAPE America to name a few.[57, 105, 106]

FitnessGram®'s approach also focuses heavily on risk modulation as a measure of long-term health, which, as previously mentioned, creates a sense of body anxiety ultimately rooted in healthism and sizeism. In an article for *Outside*, Erin Beresini expressed the concern that educational policymakers have about using measurement to determine student health in this manner.

> In the decades since Fitnessgram was first implemented, the scientific understanding of BMI's relationship to health has progressed, and American culture has changed. Instead of physical measurement, many educators and politicians have become more concerned with inclusivity and kids' mental health.[107]

The assertion that "fitness and fatness" determine health (which is only half true) is a way to play on the fear of fat and the supposed connection it bears to ill health. It is known that weight stigma is a greater risk to health, especially in children, than the diseases we often associate with fatness.[2] Again as with health, movement, physical fitness are presented as the antithesis of disease and death rather than something students can just feel good about.

New Zealand personal trainer Dillon Landi and NYC-based health/physical education teacher Carrie Safron[105] did a study of the FitnessGram's impact on the health and fitness attitudes of BIPOC and LGBTQIA+ youth in their respective regions and fields. They argue that "Such standardization of the physical education curriculum has been shown to narrow subjective experiences of young bodies to reproduce normative (gendered, racialized, sexualized, classist, ableist) ideals."[108, 109]

The FitnessGram measures ability, agility, and other fitness diagnostics along a gender binary, which reflects the idea that "For LGBTQ+ youth, this has meant that physical education as a subject works to repress nonbinary identities, regulating gender and sexuality through heteronormative practices."[110] For many students in these marginalized identities, especially multiple marginalized identities, phys ed class is the place where body policing becomes a measured, explicit part of the curriculum. This shifted in California in 2023, where conventional fitness tests were axed due to the same kinds of concerns about gender equity, ableism, and body image. California's concerns about equity, inclusivity, and mental health, at a policy level, questioning the need for body composition assessment and fitness testing in schools. The impetus for this interrogation of the school's relationship to fitness testing came after lawmakers passed the statewide Gender Recognition Act of 2017, allowing students to identify as nonbinary on state documents. The FitnessGram advisory board responded to pressure to add a set of fitness standards for nonbinary students by issuing all students reported as nonbinary with a personal score on the testing battery, but did not include them in the annual reporting, asserting in a later position paper that "results are most accurate using sex at birth, though teachers or parents could decide which gender identity would be most appropriate."[107]

This poem, published by a young person who Safron & Landi[105] met while gathering their research on the effects of the FitnessGram on youth attitudes toward fitness, reflects that student's experience of the PACER test, an endurance measure on the Fitnessgram®:

I hate the BEEP test

I hate the BEEP test
   I mean
      I don't really like it
         but
            I know it helps me

I jogged around the gym for 14 minutes
   I was so PROUD of myself
      I was also on the volleyball team then

I did bad on the PACER test
   THEY said
      YOU have to go to the weight room

BELOW average
   You failed
      I never passed
         I never passed   BEEP test

I hate the BEEP test
   By the end of the test
      I'm r a c i n g
         Don't even care when the click is coming

Going as f a s t as I can
   But it's all about p-a-c-i-n-g yourself

Every
   Single
      Beep
         Haunts
      Me

I hate the BEEP test
   In the top
      In the bottom
   The lowest

The highest
Getting teased
Feeling self-conscious
Feeling worse
Disappointed teacher
JUDGING
Survival of the FITTEST

...I hate the BEEP test
I hate it (all)
The report cards
Showing what percentile you are in
It felt kind of bad
Comparing yourself to others
I really did not like that

We do NOT learn anything
It makes you competitive
To get higher than everybody else

I don't know

I hate the BEEP test
We are really **un**fit
I look at the other people
I just want to do more than them
I look at the other people
Don't want to be the first out
Don't want to be ridiculed
We make allies
Drop out together
I look at the other people
I just want to keep going longer
There are two guys who always win
It's horrible
dropped out of PE
I was like
NO BEEP TEST ANYMORE

The poem illustrates that, though they have experience on a sports team, tests like the PACER® offer them feelings of defeat and judgment from peers and teachers. Though it may not be graded, that's not enough to stave off the sense of failure and public humiliation that even kids who move their bodies during organized team sports are made to feel: self-conscious, inadequate, and judged. The data collected about them becomes the story of who they are, individually and collectively, and defines them by what they can't do, instead of what they are capable of.[111]

The poem also reveals that what's missing from these standardized assessments is joy. School has replaced the joy of movement with the drudgery of measurement, monitoring, and body vigilance, and creates a culture of body anxiety and aversion to movement for even students who self-identify as athletes. Exercise, which sits on a hierarchy of our own cultural making, is superior to "movement" and even "fitness," which must be linked to weight loss to "count" for anything good. The erroneous assumption that fitness only exists to move us closer to thinness and away from disease, and can't just happen because it's fun, ignores the reality that weight is not an independent health risk – but most importantly, removes the joy from movement altogether.

*   *   *

The New York City Department of Education (NYCDOE) is home to more than 1,800 schools and over one million students P-12. Most of the students in both public and charter schools in the five boroughs of New York City are students of color (41.1 percent Hispanic/Latinx, 23.7 percent Black, and 16.5 percent Asian), according to their data at a glance.[112] They implement the NYC FitnessGram in all NYCDOE schools, and the NYCDOE runs its own BMI monitoring program using FitnessGram data.[107]

New York's specific role in fitness and perceptions of health for youth of color is notable for a number of reasons. It hosts an incredible number of parks, including the famous Central Park (built over a historically Black settlement known as Seneca Village).[113] Most of these parks were built in the years before, during, and immediately after the Great Depression by Robert Moses, who also believed in "clearing the slums" of mostly Black and Puerto Rican immigrants. He engaged in expensive beautification projects to build parks for the city's children, but had a notorious contempt for the poor – he often built his parks, and many bridges, tunnels, and parkways – right through their neighborhoods.[114]

The intentionally segregated urban planning models of the north make clear that racism was, and is, alive and well in the northern United States. Parks and playgrounds gave the poor working class and their children something to do, and were thought to be a way to "discipline people who were perceived as unruly and create activities for developing strength and ruggedness that reformers worried all city kids lacked."[72]

New York has the country's most boisterous BMI monitoring program, known as the Student Weight Status Category Reporting Survey.[115] Since 2010, state education law requires that fifty percent of public schools in New York conduct surveys annually, with the option to opt students out at a district level. The data collected has revealed that "obesity" is low among elementary school students, but rising in middle and high school students. Could this be from things such as standardized testing, the pressure to look to the future instead of remaining in the present, and the allostatic load (the body's physiological "wear and tear" as a response to stressors) brought on by school as children go through the K-12 system? The "public health opportunity" suggestions presented in this data set are more time for physical activity and more access to water in place of sugary beverages at school.[116] But what about less academic pressure and stress?

This data has also reflected that "obesity" is rising in "high needs" districts. In education, "high needs" is synonymous with districts who have a high percentage of students who live below the poverty line, chronic issues retaining teachers, or have one or more teachers teaching out of their content area.[117, 118] This is also coded language for schools with high incidences of poverty, populations with large numbers of BIPOC students and families, or a combination of both. Many schools considered "high needs" have a high population of students utilizing free and reduced lunch programs. Additionally, this label becomes another way of saying that "high needs" means "at risk" (of what, exactly?) and thus, these communities need to be monitored, further educated, and "saved" by the institutions who "know better." The conclusion drawn by 2013 reports on "high needs" districts is that school districts with a high incidence of students on free and reduced lunch programs are "priority settings for obesity prevention programs."[51] The term "at-risk youth" is thrown around and placed adjacent to youth of color in ways similarly coded to "high needs," including in the realm of physical education. People in power profile youth of color for the many risks they supposedly carry – to themselves, to others, to their environment – since time immemorial. Mike Brown, Tamir Rice, and other Black youth (Chapter 2) have been categorized as "threatening" for not only their Blackness, but also the size of their bodies. In health and physical education, they do not escape this trope, either. Except in phys ed or health class, they are seen as a risk to themselves and their broader cultural community.

According to the NYC Department of Education,

> NYC FITNESSGRAM is an annual fitness assessment for students in grades kindergarten-twelve that helps students and their families develop personal goals for lifelong fitness. Students complete the assessments in Physical Education class. NYC FITNESSGRAM is not a graded test, and the results are confidential.[119]

This aligns with the FitnessGram advisory board's recommendations, the NYC FitnessGram is not graded, so the pressure of a score that goes in the gradebook is absent. This is especially good news for students whose PE grade is tied to their ability to graduate, as is the case for students in New York. The results are confidential; so no one will see the numbers – the BMI, the number of laps run, etc. In most cases, though, the test is administered publicly, meaning that peers are there to watch you try, and maybe even fail.

FitnessGram® attempts to ease criticism about these very real anxieties created by their body composition assessment by saying there is "no research evidence" that body composition assessments in general "will make a child overly concerned about their body and lead to eating disorders."[33] It also appears to be race and class neutral, though its media and promotional materials clearly target specific populations. Karisa Butler-Wall analyzed a 2011 promotional video in which an African American mother "becomes the main spokesperson for the power of FitnessGram to change the lifestyles of children at school."[57] This promotional video typecasts Black mothers in particular, and families of color in general, as ignorant to their child's health and fitness status: and by "representing parental ignorance as the source of childhood obesity, this video participates in a larger cultural narrative suggesting that working-class women of color lack proper information about health and fitness."[57]

FitnessGram plays a major role in a large-scale, systematic effort to improve the health and wellness outcomes of youth, specifically youth of color, at a federal level. It has become absorbed into today's iteration of the Presidential Council on Youth Fitness. The program is a small piece of the larger puzzle that is former First Lady Michelle Obama's *Let's Move!* Campaign. For her years as First Lady (and beyond), the initiative has targeted schools, media, and other access points to get young people to move more as a response to ending "childhood obesity."

Butler-Wall argues in her paper that *"Let's Move! Reinforces cultural associations between obesity, poverty and racialized populations."*[57] It engages in the doublespeak of making the "childhood obesity crisis" both a universal and individual problem, by creating an issue around the very real health disparities among racialized populations. Obama's website is quick to point out that 40 percent of Black and Hispanic children in America are overweight, and that

> If we don't solve this problem, one third of all children born in 2000 or later will have diabetes at some point in their lives. Many others will face chronic obesity-related health problems like heart disease, high blood pressure, cancer, and asthma.[120]

Rhetoric such as this fossilizes in the American consciousness that "race stands in as a proxy for the likelihood of obesity and ill health." The larger narrative does not address the larger problems – industrialized, obesogenic environments,[121] race, class, and gender inequality, school lunch debt, clean air and water, green space privilege, etc. – and instead makes all of these things a matter of individual education that parents and kids supposedly lack.

In reality what they lack is control over their ability to change the conditions that policies and politics have created. Since *Let's Move!*, temporary and part-time labor has increased in the United States, combined with the expansion of the fast food industry through government subsidies.[33] Access to healthy food isn't a matter of ignorance, or even tangible availability; it's a matter of affordability and structural equity.

This imagery echoes the Progressive era reformer idea that Black, Brown, and poor bodies needed to be controlled, monitored, and "disciplined," because they had nothing to do (because they were not permitted to attend safe schools due to racism) and "didn't know better" – suggesting a superiority that of course, neoliberal progressives, had the answer to. Thus, they "gifted" them parks and playgrounds, but backhanded them with rising housing costs and no meaningful way out of poverty. This pattern continues beyond the *Let's Move!* campaign.

After NYC FitnessGram® testing is done, parents receive a colorful, chart-laden report about their child's results, available to them in print and digital formats in nine different languages. It presents to them data on a child's weight and height only in grades K-3; a BMI report card, more or less. In the higher grades, students are measured for height and weight, and evaluated additionally on five activities assessing their "strength, endurance, flexibility and aerobic capacity."[119] The NYCDOE website invites families with questions about their students' report to contact their child's physical education teacher to find out more about how the test was administered, what the results mean, and "how your student can make a plan to stay healthy and fit."

When considering who the majority of these report recipients are – largely Black and Brown, and many, mostly low-income students and their families – it brings to light the reality that "Black and Latinx youth may come to find their bodies at odds with a standardized practice that disregards their own race and culture."[122] In their critical analysis of the program, Saffron & Landi explain that

> As a system rooted in Westernized biomedical measures, FitnessGram® can exacerbate such 'at-risk' and deficit perspectives. Its health-related practices (e.g. Progressive Aerobic Cardiovascular Endurance Run (PACER), body composition) continues to be centered around white (often masculine) physiological markers of the body. Such approaches reinforce a narrative that Black and Latinx families are in need of intervention regarding their lifestyles, erasing broader cultural, social, economic, and political considerations.[105]

NYCDOE's page on Physical Education curriculum says, "These Healthy Fitness Zone standards represent a level of fitness that offers some degree of protection against health problems associated with physical inactivity. Students are not compared to each other or to a fixed norm."[123] However, BMI is used in this score report, and it is, by definition, a fixed norm (based on white, middle-aged, male bodies).

FitnessGram prides itself on forty years of research and the development of the first "fitness report card." In the years since, BMI report cards are now required in 25 American states.[17] Despite body mass index not being a reliable measure of health, even in its early conception, it is still used as a proxy for student fitness levels and as a judgment of their overall physical well-being. In a randomized controlled study in 79 California schools, researchers followed students from grades 3–8 who received BMI report cards and found that no change was made in their overall body composition or weight status during that time; but their attempts at unhealthy weight control as well as their body dissatisfaction increased.[124] So, not only are these report cards ineffective at the job they sought out to do of monitoring student "health" data to "motivate" them to stay in shape, they actually make students feel worse about their bodies, which is known to drive them *away* from physical activity and healthful eating. Instead, policymakers and educators worry tools like BMI report cards increase weight stigma, familial blame, and fat shaming among the kids and families who receive them.

The Center for Disease Control (CDC) makes no specific recommendations or policy about how student health data such as BMI is to be collected in schools. Despite it being seen as a method of "tackling" the "childhood obesity epidemic," BMI data collection has been found not to reduce size or weight status in American children. The current CDC guidance states that it "does not make a recommendation for or against BMI measurement programs in schools. It does suggest that schools create 'safe, supportive environments for students of all body sizes', 'a comprehensive set of strategies to prevent and reduce obesity', and 'a series of safeguards that address the primary concerns raised about such programs'."[125] What's contradictory about these suggestions is that there doesn't really seem to be any equitable or just way to "create a safe space for all body sizes" if you're going to, in the same breath, suggest that the people in larger body sizes are intrinsically wrong and should be prevented and "reduced." This dichotomy comes with the inherent suggestion that there is a "right" way to be in a body, and "safeguarding" the process of tracking student's weight as a stand-in for their health feels, well, counterintuitive.

In their guidelines, the CDC says that

> to date, there is not enough evidence for scientists to con-clude whether school-based BMI measurement programs are effective at preventing or reducing childhood obesity or whether they cause harm, by either increasing the stigma attached to obesity or increasing pressures to engage in unsafe weight control behaviors;[125]

thus, the CDC undercuts the need for BMI measurement in schools but still stands by their implementation. The same statement advises educators that "before implementing these programs, decision makers need to consider the costs involved, potential negative consequences for students, and existing school-based strategies to support healthy weight-related behaviors and prevent weight-based bullying." They list ten safeguarding recommendations, which are, in short: (1) informed consent with families (2) appropriate staff training (3) maintaining confidentiality (4) reliable measurement and equipment (5) correct BMI calculation (6) sufficient staff to efficiently collect data (7) not using data as a basis for grading or teacher evaluation (8) assess the process, including intended and unintended consequences of the program. (9) follow up (10) provide parents with clear, respectful follow up, and prognosis.[125]

What happens instead is a mark of shame upon their bodies and their families (who are blamed for "not caring for them," as with the Regino family mentioned in Chapter 1). If the argument is that families need to know things about their children's health, BMI is certainly not an accurate or reliable place to start. It is hard not to see how the narrative of an "epidemic" and the need to avoid weight stigma are inherently contradictory; and this contradiction is being made plain even by the government agencies and officials invested in perpetuating the idea that fatness is a "killer disease."[126]

A lot of these safeguards go against the exact messaging they're aiming to promote, similar to the diet industry co-opting the language of body positivity. What good is correct BMI calculation, if the medical community and society have expressed doubt that BMI isn't an accurate or reliable measure of health? If it's not a reliable measure of student health, why would we use it against teachers? Why would we use it to determine anything about a student, or their physical health, or their phys ed teacher's effectiveness at teaching them about their health, at all? If the implication of an "unintended consequence" of collecting BMI data from students might be weight and body dissatisfaction, why risk collecting this information from kids whose self-concept is already developmentally fragile?

The intention and care given to health and wellness gets lost among the decades of bad science, bad data, and assumptions-as-policy it is built on. Initiatives predicated on the idea that kids' bodies are a problem, and the parents doing what they can with the resources they can are at fault, is not one that aims to create collaborative, lasting partnerships invested in health. Instead, it crafts policy and curriculum on the assumptions that (a) fat bodies are not healthy, (b) that fat people aren't and don't know how to take care of themselves, and (c) that the built environment, systematic oppression, and variable access to social determinants of health can they can be repaired through individual actions. Physical education curriculum that does not address things like access to nutrient dense food, safe space to play, and movement that is adaptive and responsive to all bodies is not going to set students up to "develop personal goals for lifelong fitness." It will, and it does, instead, set them up to develop personal feelings of lifelong shame, guilt, and anxiety around food and movement. Four veteran physical educators: Chris Ehlert, Rip Marston, Fabio Fontana, and Jennifer Waldron offer concrete advice to reframe physical education for students in larger bodies, beginning with changing language that disarms implicit bias and assumptions about what physical activity students are capable of. They suggest that teachers' perceptions of students who slow down in an activity or exercise as "lazy" or "unmotivated" can lead to interactions that reveal bias on behalf of the teacher, regardless of the intention. This can lead to students feeling less confident and likely to engage in physical education class and, over time, in physical activity as a whole. "In reality, the student's heart rate may be above the workout zone," they said. They suggest reframing and validating students' efforts, adding, "If the teacher announces, 'Get going' or 'You are not working hard,'" the student may react negatively and shut down. If, instead, the teacher approaches the student and asks, "How are you feeling?" or "Have you checked your heart rate?"[127] The latter approach helps students to be more attuned to their body's needs, and gives them permission to listen to what that body is telling them, rather than performing activity beyond their threshold or spiraling into self-comparing against their peers.

The goal of connecting schools, families, and healthcare providers to student health also falls apart when those same students are seeing diminishing access to clean air and green spaces, decreasing access to public spaces such as libraries, malls, and places to socialize, an increase in student anxiety and inability to self-regulate, and a decrease in program funding via austerity budgets. Without acknowledging the network of overlapping and underlying issues, all that remains is a "fitness program" purported by a system that, as usual, puts the onus on individual kids and their families for maintaining their overall health and wellness in a political and social climate that often prioritizes neither.

*   *   *

Using BMI report cards and other tracking and monitoring tools to measure students' longitudinal health outcomes is a part of FitnessGram®'s model, which under the Obama Administration was slated to be implemented in 90 percent of U.S. public schools by 2018 – with ten million dollars from General Mills to make it happen.[57] Using children's data as a tool (and as a product) poses many issues for long-term health and the potential for compulsive body monitoring that lasts a lifetime, as well as for the privacy of their personally identifiable information as well. "The obesity epidemic has engendered new measures of control that operate through a logic of preemption, constituting new populations for intervention according to a racialized calculus of risk."[57] The FitnessGram model of assessing students' risk factors by collecting their demographic information leaves room for a lot of generalizations about culture, family, and social determinants of health to be negatively levied against students. It also leaves room for cultural assumptions, generalizations, and eugenicist myths to take shape around Black and Brown bodies, placing them in a category of risk based on "objective criterion based standards."[33] But these criteria appear to be a cluster of assumptions based on race, location, self-reported physical activity, and calculated BMI; with no mention of genetics, which play the largest role in physical and overall health.[75] The system designates students who fall below the Healthy Fitness Zone for their age and gender categories are designated as "Needs Improvement," and informed that they carry a category indicating a "potential for future health risks."[57] While it's true that lack of movement contributes greatly to the presence of disease regardless of a person's weight[19] the idea of "needs improvement" and scaring students with potential health risks they haven't met yet does not seem like a motivator to get, and stay, fit. In fact, things like healthism and stigma toward fatness make people generally "more likely to avoid exercise, regardless of actual Body Mass Index."[3] Being told your body "needs improvement" does not seem like the best way to forge a positive relationship with that body. Students who feel less capable are more likely to give up on movement altogether. If we want students to fear their bodies less and move more, a lifetime of constant monitoring may not be the way to go. Health curriculums should focus more comprehensively on eating disorder prevention and explicitly discussing weight stigma with students, since it is more likely to negatively impact their health than high weight – in both the long and short term.

Big Moves for Physical Education Teachers and Administrators

♦ Show images of bodies in all sizes and shapes engaging in movement they like.

♦ Get to know your students' movement habits and family movement habits without judgment or shame.

♦ Make movement and fitness about how students feel, not about how they look. If you can, remove mirrors from physical activity spaces to discourage hypervigilance and self-monitoring based on appearance.

♦ Talk to students about limit-setting around exercise and movement, and knowing when their body is tired and should rest.

♦ Hire people of all identities, shapes, sizes, and abilities to teach health and physical education.

♦ Help students develop a relationship with movement that is free from diet talk, weight loss, or reduction mindsets; encourage them to find movement that they enjoy doing, without pressure to track or log it.

♦ Find activities that work for everyone – I personally was SO bad at team sports as a neurodivergent person, but I loved track and cross country because it was independent and the only person I was up against was myself.

♦ Have students build assessments and success criteria with you so that everyone can meet their goals instead of focusing heavily on skill.

♦ Ask administrators or community members for help getting adaptive equipment such as yoga blocks, bolsters, and cushions so that students at all fitness levels can participate comfortably.

From the Ashes, A Paradigm Shift

If health is truly a priority in our schools, why not make health education last their entire school experience, so that they can learn more intricately about the social determinants of health, about the role of genes, calories, movement, hormones, and body composition, and about nutrition; instead of just playing *Supersize Me!*? When I was in high school, health class happened in tenth grade, every other day, for just a semester. I argue that in order to do better, and give students a curriculum that is more in depth, they need more time in health class with teachers who are given consistent, informed guidelines about *all* the factors that contribute to health. The less comprehensive our health curriculums are, the more weight stigma they are apt to perpetuate. We need more frequent and greater in-depth health education that is accessible to all, and focuses on personal and collective definitions and behaviors that make up overall health. Schools also must consider developing a policy that minimizes competition and comparison among students and their physical fitness abilities, even if the comparisons are only happening socially and not for a grade. Environments where everyone isn't just welcome, but is encouraged to participate and show up as they are, make a difference in the lifelong habits of all students.

As with any practice of diversity, equity, inclusion, and belonging, we must do more than merely *state* that we accept all bodies in physical education and fitness spaces. The people who need that acceptance the most must *feel* that belonging and acceptance, if we are to call our physical education programs successfully inclusive.

> Most medical and government health recommendations (not to mention innumerable corporate initiatives ad campaigns and even reality TV shows) focus on the need for individual change to improve public health, when what's really needed if people are to live better and longer is social change.[75]

One solution to the rugged individualism (and body shame) that physical education has cultivated in the minds and bodies of American kids lies in what Bacon & Aphramor call *active embodiment*.[75] Born of principles of Health at Every Size (HAES), active embodiment encourages people in all bodies to "engage in physical activity that is enjoyable, healthy, and sustainable."[1] HAES "supports people of all sizes in addressing health directly by adopting healthy behaviors" and includes "respect, critical awareness, and compassionate self-care."[4, 128] If we are going to commit to change, we must change our commitments. In reimagining health and physical education curriculum, several considerations are paramount: ending size and weight as a stand-in for our definitions of health, expanding that understanding outward, creating anti-bullying and curriculum development policy that explicitly states the inherent worth of people in all sized bodies and acknowledges natural size diversity; changing our language and practice to reflect our commitment to that policy, and ongoing feedback loops about how these changes impact those they benefit – teachers and students in larger bodies.

HAES, a framework created in the 1990s by the Association for Size Diversity and Health, has four key principles: (1) that healthcare is a human right for people of all sizes, including those at the highest end of the size spectrum. (2) Wellbeing, care, and healing are resources that are both collective and deeply personal. (3) Care is fully provided only when free from anti-fat bias and offered with people of all sizes in mind. (4) Health is a socio-political construct that reflects the values of society. Their framework rests upon these principles, and includes values of liberation, consent, autonomy, compassion, and freedom from oppression.[129] HAES calls upon us as a culture to see body image, health, access to care, and an end to weight bias as a social justice issue, and to act accordingly.

In March of 2025, Dr. Mehmet Oz, known mostly for his daytime TV show, declared that it is one's "patriotic duty to be healthy,"[130] so that they can become part of the military-industrial complex. He serves as the overseer of Medicare and Medicaid, after a long career of platforming debunked science, especially that about fatness and obesity.

For both of these public officials that health is predicated on one's productivity and ability to support the war machine seems to be a running thesis of their understanding and framing of health. When this is the case, peoples' value lies solely in their bodies being able to contribute to the mission of a state that seeks to oppress or eliminate them if they aren't.

Critics of fat acceptance frequently misread the acronym as meaning "health at ANY size," which is incorrect and misrepresents the full scope of the framework. "HAES does not claim that everyone is at a healthy weight. What it does is ask for respect and help people shift their focus away from changing their size to enhancing their self-care behaviors."[19] The same critics are ones who are most likely to view fatness as self-inflicted and fatness as unacceptable, unattractive, and unhealthy.[131] Media representations such as *My 600 Pound Life* and *1000 Pound Sisters*, a show that caricatures and sensationalizes very fat bodies, make these criticisms and biases more concrete. These fat bodies represent fewer than two percent of the human population, but are made to look like the rule rather than the exception. This is a moment for teaching media literacy and criticality; one that we will cover more extensively in Chapter 4.

Believe it or not, this chapter is the condensed version of how these ideas intersect to frame our understanding of health. From here, we will apply what we've learned about how we arrived at this moment to other areas of school as we know them. Ultimately, the hope is that a HAES-inspired framework and safer, more equitable and welcoming physical activity spaces in schools will inspire students to feel less likely to resent physical activity into adulthood. Here are a few ideas for making that happen:

RUN IT BACK: Reflecting on Your Practice

♦ *Assess your own relationship to movement; is it joyful, compensatory, fraught, or some combination of things?*

♦ *How can you help students improve their relationship with movement away from diet culture and in the direction of joy?*

♦ *How can you make joyful movement a part of your classroom practice, regardless of content area?*

♦ *What kinds of conversations does your school have with students and families about health and wellness? Are there cultural, gendered, or other assumptions built into these conversations that need to be interrogated?*

II

Hit Pause

The chapters in Part II of this book will offer strategies for how we can pause the biases we see and hear happening so that we can shuffle into a more equitable future.

DOI: 10.4324/9781003534143-6

5

The Miseducation of Everyone

Weight Stigma across Content Areas

The NYU Metro Center defines curriculum as "the detailed package of learning goals; units, and lessons that lay out what teachers teach each day and week assignments, activities, and projects given to students; and books, materials, videos, presentations and readings used in the class."[11] The incomplete story about fat that we're selling to kids in the form of science, math, health, nutrition, and literacy curriculum points to the need for more conversation between content areas and a shared commitment to ending diet culture. With so much content to teach, and an average mandate of 180 days to teach it, getting entire schools on board and engaging in the work of unlearning is a necessary and important step to the rule of "first do no harm."

Often associated with doctors, the first job we have is trying our hardest to do no harm in the classroom. It is entirely possible, and necessary, to be on our own growth and unlearning journey in the process – and diet culture and white supremacy culture want us to believe that we have to get it perfect before we can deliver the kinds of equity we hope to achieve to kids. But here, perfectionism will not deliver progress. In Part I, we unmasked diet culture myths, and we'll keep at it; but in this part, we'll cover all the ways that "first do no harm" remains our responsibility,

DOI: 10.4324/9781003534143-7

and harness the power that we have as experts in our content to fulfill that responsibility in our teaching. Seeing our content areas as separate entities, blocks of time, or standalone strands of ideas or packaged units is how we miss the ways that fatphobia and its close relatives, racism, ableism, xenophobia, queerphobia, and white supremacy – show up in the content we transmit to students. Integration of ideas, noticing and seeing patterns, and never forgetting that everything is interconnected is how we suffocate the systems that harm.

Just Eat It

One subject that affects so many of the others in a school setting is our knowledge (or lack thereof, really) of nutrition and the body. Our perception of food, our physical appearance, and ourselves permeates all that we do, and for kids especially, their ability to learn. Most American students who have received nutrition education in the last six decades can remember some iteration of geometry explaining what, and how much, we should eat daily. From FDR to JFK to *Let's Move!*, American nutrition guidelines, like physical education programs, have always been politically motivated before they were scientific. Nutrition science actually wasn't much of a priority in the federal government until the mid-20th century, when the U.S. Department of Agriculture (USDA) explored the relationships between urbanization, rural farmers, and agricultural growth. Milk and produce were luxuries, especially between wars, and valued for the ways that they protected against diseases like rickets and scurvy. Perhaps an explanation for Bonnie Prudden's findings a decade later, it was discovered by 1940 that 40 percent of WWII recruits were deemed unfit to serve because they were underweight or malnourished. As we entered a second global war, the state of our fighting men just wouldn't cut it; leading President Roosevelt to consider nutrition a problem of national magnitude, enough to begin studying it more closely. This query would lead to what we know today as the USDA's national school lunch program, and the first iteration of Supplemental Nutrition Assistance

Program (SNAP), colloquially known by many Americans as food stamps.[132]

The food pyramid is actually an invention of the Swedish, created in the 1970s and adapted by the USDA in 1992.[133] The USDA revised it again in 2005 to MyPyramid, a more personalized and updated version based on agricultural availability and changes in American diet patterns. It was again replaced by the MyPlate model in 2011. Is your head spinning yet?

All this geometry representing what "should" be our diet doesn't originate in any nutrition or dietary science at all. In both Sweden and America, the creation of dietary guidelines arose as a response to U.S. wartime food shortages in 1943 and rising food costs in Sweden in 1970.[133] The USDA divided food into seven basic groups; among them are bread and cereals, fruits and vegetables, meat and poultry. The 1992 version included four levels, containing serving recommendations and daily reference values for each group: breads, cereals, rice, and pasta (6–11 servings daily); vegetables (3–5 servings daily; fruits (2–4 servings daily) dairy (2–3 servings daily); meat, poultry, and fish (2–3 servings daily); and fats and oils (sparingly).

In fact, the 2,000-calorie diet doesn't come rooted in any medical or scientific basis. Instead, the Food and Drug Administration (FDA) recommended this calorie amount and percent daily values on Americans' self-reported calorie intakes, which ranged from 1,600 to 3,000 calories per day.[134] They initially recommended 2,350, but feared this would encourage overeating, so they rounded it down.[135] To make it even more imprecise and confusing, food manufacturers are legally allowed to misrepresent that information, too. In the United States, regulations permit nutrition labels to reflect up to a 20 percent margin of error.[75] So how can we expect to use nutrition labeling reliably as a measure of our health if the goalposts are constantly moving?

Critics of food pyramids and other similar guidelines say that the food pyramid oversimplifies the notion of the ideal diet, and does little to educate people on the varying nutrient profiles of the foods in each group.[133] The guidelines changed again when in 2005, the original template was said to be blamed in connection to the obesity epidemic, because the recommended serving of carbohydrates did not differentiate between simple and complex carbs, which serve different nutritional roles and different types of fats, which differ in function and nutritional necessity as well. The current MyPlate guidelines, created in 2011, offer instead a more visual to-scale model of what the average person's plate should look like; and what food groups (and how much of them) to include on the plate at each meal.[133]

In an article for *CNN*, body image parent coach Oona Hanson notes that

> Children across all grade levels are taught nutrition concepts aimed at improving health, but I find these well-intended lessons can end up backfiring, harming kids' eating habits and their overall well-being. Nutrition lessons – largely driven by state education standards – can be damaging because they unintentionally convey the same messages as an eating disorder: cut out certain foods, limit calories and fear weight gain.[136]

Health curriculum is increasingly skills-based, and one of those skills is often reading nutrition labels and making decisions about what to eat. Hanson interviewed several nutrition experts and dietitians, who noted that many lessons, which ask students to categorize foods as "good" or "bad" can carry implicit messaging that eating certain foods and not others equates to them being "good" or "bad." Food is morally neutral, and language that calls food "junk" or "garbage" will not help the ever-increasing body dissatisfaction our students are already feeling.[137]

Dr. Taylor Arnold, a registered dietitian and "kid nutrition expert" has some phenomenal suggestions on her Instagram page @growing.intuitive.eaters for parents, teachers, and adults who work with kids to help them learn about their bodies and food in a neutral-positive light that has been lacking in nutrition curriculum. She is also the mom of a preschooler, and regularly teaches nutrition lessons to her kids' classes that help them learn about food in ways that she says can happen "without calling any foods bad, or using "healthy vs. unhealthy" worksheets."[138] During one lesson on citrus fruits with four year olds, she brought in slices of oranges, lemons, limes and grapefruits – and had students make inferences about how the fruit would look once it was cut open, what it would smell like, and whether slices of it would sink or float with or without the peel. They also discussed using a visual map of the body where the citrus goes in the body once it's eaten. This age-appropriate way of exploring food is a fantastic way to incorporate sensory learning, curiosity, and inquiry, and a morally neutral approach to food.

For middle and high school nutrition education, she offers a list of suggestions in another post for reframing and rethinking nutrition education, including suggestions like teaching cooking skills, "easy, no-cook options to fuel your body, eating on a budget, how to build a plate to fuel your mental health and physical health, eating disorder prevention, and the influence of diet culture, what are fiber, carbs, protein, fat, and where do you find them?; How to fuel your body for physical activity (and not just for student athletes!)" She also emphasizes risk reduction: talking about alcohol, diet scams, detoxes, energy drinks, supplements, and diet myths. She also notes that she intentionally does not include calorie counting on this list, because she argues, "we don't need to teach teens that."[139]

Get the FACs

Many FACS programs now teach more culinary skills, sustainability, the concept of "slow foods," and appreciation for local agriculture like the kind Dr. Arnold advocates for in her videos. This is a positive step in the right direction, but it's only one subject.

At the school where I teach, students have even learned and focused their quarter in FACS class on the United Nations Sustainable Development Goals, which echo many of the tenets of the social determinants of health. These curricular shifts offer opportunities for students to learn about indigenous agricultural traditions, target food waste locally in their school, and more. The addition of these goals into the FACS curriculum facilitates conversation between multiple genres and subject areas – media literacy, health, science, and social studies to name just a few.

Programs like the Berkeley Edible Schoolyard Project encourage students to grow, cook, and taste food together, which can empower them to know what's in their food and engage in the process of community building while gaining lifelong independence and culinary skills. Their mission statement conveys their dedication "to the transformation of public education by using organic school gardens, kitchens, and cafeterias to teach both academic subjects and the values of nourishment, stewardship, and community."[140] Other teaching tools like Nourish and Cooking with Curiosity provide materials, lessons, and videos that are adaptive to students of all ages and can help frame conversations around food that are free from diet culture.

FACs class is also an opportunity to teach students about how to critically read a nutrition label and be smarter consumers. Many agencies such as the USDA, FDA, and World Health Organization (WHO) dictate the standard of what is permitted to make it onto our plates. Everything we've been taught about nutrition at school has largely been the effort of these agencies. "Calorie counts and labels, it seems, have always been shaped by social anxieties about fatness," argues Aubrey Gordon.[17] As my friend Liz pointed out earlier in this chapter, calories don't have to be the enemy; especially not for students whose bodies are growing through puberty and changing all the time. Combating misinformation and the public enemy status of food and eating is a mammoth mission, but it is a mission: possible with the right combination of teachers committed to actively unlearning anti-fat biases and the intention to help heal our students' relationship to food and body image alongside our own.

One content creator doing the work of unraveling anti-fat pseudoscience is Dr. Jess Steier, critic of the "food infodemic" of misinformation and fear mongering around food. In an August 2024 post, she debunks another creator's infographic about chicken nuggets, a common "competitive food" in student cafeterias across America. In the post, she addresses the food science of the most vilified chicken nugget in America: McDonald's. She says "While this post isn't an endorsement of frequent fast food consumption, it aims to debunk misinformation, correct false claims, and alleviate unwarranted anxiety about occasionally eating these nuggets as part of a balanced diet."[141] In the original post, the creator who problematizes McNuggets suggests that "dimethylpolysiloxane, a perfectly safe anti-foaming agent used in various foods," is the same ingredient used in silly putty.

Dr. Steier points out that "just because a substance is used in two different products doesn't mean it has the same function or safety profile in both."[141] She also notes that this compound is "not readily absorbed in the gastrointestinal tract, with the vast majority excreted unchanged in feces." She even does the math to address overblown claims, saying that "the average person would need to consume 756 chicken nuggets in one day for this to be considered a potential concern."[141] One of the biggest mistakes we make is immediately associating "chemicals" and "processed" with negative health outcomes, when in fact, chemicals and chemistry exist in the natural world all around us. Being critical of the ways that these compounds function is a type of scientific literacy grounded in spotting and demystifying food-related logical fallacies.

"When will I use this in real life?"

It feels important to note that our cultural perception of weight and health, in the first place, has everything to do with just three things: fear, politics, and math. The health, diet, and medical industrial complex have worked together for decades to alert us to an epidemic; one whose fears that they promised would lead to lower rates of longevity and worse health outcomes for the sole sin of being fat, has yet to materialize. Paul Campos states:

> Our latest surge of panic over what by now must surely be the longest running "epidemic" in medical history is largely a product of statistical manipulation. Because the population's weight follows a standard distribution (bell curve), placing the definition for overweight and obese near the population's median for weight guarantees that an average weight increase of just a few pounds will

suddenly throw millions of Americans in the overweight and obese categories.[34]

It also feels important to frame for teachers that we cannot divorce our students' understanding of math, statistics, and probability from constantly changing political and cultural motivations. These biases show up in our word problems, our questioning, and our assumptions about what students know and can do, every day and in every way.

I found a video on YouTube called "Using MATH to LOSE WEIGHT!" by a channel called Teach Me Animated Math. In just eight minutes, it shows the audience how to apply knowledge of polynomials (an eighth-grade math skill) to calculate what a person would need to lose weight for their body. The idea of students having access to this information is scary, especially for eighth graders who are already wrestling with all the ways they believe their bodies need fixing coupled with their developing sense of self and self-esteem. When we think about all the ways that we hope kids will apply their mathematical knowledge in real life, this kind of information feels like a roadmap to compulsive counting and compensatory behavior. When I was in my WiiFit era as a middle schooler, I wasn't quite savvy enough to use polynomials to calculate my BMR or energy balance equation; but I certainly knew what both of those were, and had a spreadsheet do it for me. In my years as a teacher, I have seen and heard questions posed to students asking them to calculate the "number of pounds someone would need to lose…" and other such framing.

In a section about math and science, it seems important to mention that they noted what researcher John Robison found: that in relation to other conditions such as autism, cerebral palsy, Down syndrome, sudden infant death syndrome (SIDS) cancer, only 12 incidences of type 2 diabetes per 100,000 children were found. "This means," Bacon and Aphramour explain, "that a child is 242 times more likely to have an eating disorder than type 2 diabetes."[75] Consider this an invitation to teach students the importance of not only collecting and interpreting data, but also differentiating relationships between data sets.

Many teacher pages circulate a popular photo for a laugh that presents a math question with a snarky answer supposedly written by a student. The paper in the photo reads: "Bob has 36 candy bars. He eats 29. What does he have now?" to which the respondent answered "Diabetes. Bob has diabetes."[142] There are many iterations of this joke on the internet, meant to make people laugh; but what's really happening is that they're using math for likes and reactions, and laughing at Bob, a hypothetical overeater who, according to the punchline, got diabetes solely from eating 29 candy bars. "Jokes" like this make the link between fatphobia and healthism concrete. This may seem like a one-off, cheeky answer to a question that lives only as a meme, but real-world problems that ask students to calculate the ratio of chips and candy someone eats to how fat they get perpetuates the stereotype that all fat people binge eat.[18] It's very mathematical, actually, to see people as more than parts of who they are – fat people are whole people.

Lindo Bacon and Lucy Aphramor unpack these stereotypes in *Body Respect*. To address the assertion that America's kids are getting fatter, they cite the National Health and Nutrition Examination Survey, which indicates that American kids' weights have been relatively stable since 1999; and that there is no data supporting the common media assertion that today's kids will have shorter lives than those of their parents.[75] A common concern about American children is their supposed propensity toward diabetes. In the past decade, the commercial featuring Wilford Brimley has become a meme, and fodder for fatphobic jokes about too much sugar or being overweight. Bacon and Aphramor debunk this myth of a rise in type 2 diabetes in children; citing a study published in the *Journal of the American Medical Association*, they discuss findings that reveal that type 2 diabetes – the kind often associated with insulin resistance and "obesity" – is exceptionally rare in children and virtually non-existent in kids under age ten.[75]

Understanding that correlation and causation are two different statistical items is the work of a good mathematician. As I've repeated for emphasis throughout the text, weight is not by itself an indicator of poor health or a risk of disease. However, fat people can get sick just like thin people can – and while size may be *related* to certain conditions, being fat does not affirmatively *cause* or even guarantee them – It's important that we, and our students, know the difference. When we transmit this understanding, it makes it possible to teach students that their bodies are not something to fear, and creates a learning space where stereotypes, microaggressions, and jokes about fat bodies like "Bob has diabetes" are not acceptable. It also makes the work of integrating their understanding of science, health, physical education, and embodiment much, much easier.

Math is all about solving problems; not just the numerical kind. Inviting students to ask questions that lead to conversation about weight stigma, size acceptance, food access, and how to make school a better place for everyone in all of these areas. Take the figures that have been widely accepted as fact and break them down mathematically.

Sample Calculation Questions for Students:

- ◆ What is methodology? How is methodology used to interpret data?
- ◆ What percentage of students in our community live in a food desert?
- ◆ How much physical activity do students at our school do each week?
- ◆ How many students feel hungry before vs. after their lunch period?

These questions empower students to come up with solutions to problems, form hypotheses about them, and investigate their thinking; and along the way, teachers can model how to interpret the information they find.

Quick Tip

The overlap in studying data and critical media consumption is a great opportunity to collaborate across curriculum. Teachers in science, FACS, math, and beyond can plan lessons together that encourage students to look more closely at popular data and statistics, trends, and social phenomena from a mathematical lens.

Follow the Money

As we've learned from various pandemics, vaccine debates, and more, science is hardly ever free from political influence. The science connecting health, nutrition, and weight is no different. Science class through the lens of weight stigma can teach students how to read statistics, look critically at labels, question the framing of information presented to them, test theories for themselves, and make sense of research – including research that is motivated not by science, but bias.

In his book *The Obesity Myth*, Paul Campos cites the ways that researchers present data, and then draw conclusions that do not draw a linear trajectory from their own description of their data: the "300,000 people per year die from being obese" generalization is one such case.[34] The study often connected to this statistic, published in the *Journal of the American Medical Association* as a "fact," says in its methodology: "Our calculations assume that all (controlling for age, sex and smoking) excess mortality in obese people is due to their adiposity."[34] So, controlling for basically three factors that are related to health outcomes, including one that is causally related to premature death and disease (smoking?).

This statistic and the rhetoric created around it are still commonly used to raise an alarm about the "obesity epidemic" in America and in classrooms. In a critique of the study, Campos indicates the researchers do not investigate the relationship between dietary content, lifestyle, use of diet drugs, socioeconomic status, healthcare access, or other social determinants that accounted for some or all of the excess mortality they observed among fat participants.[34] In short, the data collected tells only part of the story of the health profiles of the people it claims are most likely to die of obesity related deaths. Painting half the picture in the name of potential financial interest is unscientific at best and dangerous at worst.

Dr. Charles Hennekens, a medical researcher and consultant for the FDA, is quoted in *New York Times* saying "Epidemiology is a crude and inexact science...we tend to overstate findings, either because we want attention or more grant money."[143] Scientific inquiry is a process of finding answers to concrete and abstract questions, and can also invite us to think: "What's the story?" As an ELA teacher, I often ask my students to think critically about who is telling a story; what their motivations are for telling a story; and pay attention to the author's use of certain details, as well as the choice to leave them out. We must teach these same critical thinking skills in science, where unfortunately, research about weight (and the conclusions that the researchers draw) is often not free of this need for criticality. Making the connections between politics, policy, profit and science is one way that students can continue to question the ethics and outcomes of the science they encounter. The NIH, WHO, and other agencies consider "obesity experts," for instance, to be people who run weight loss clinics – that is, those with a vested monetary interest in people pursuing weight loss, even in the absence of empirical evidence that weight loss is necessary for health.

Susan Wooley refers to this as the "P.S. Phenomenon," as in "P.S.: Fund me again" – a coded message from the researcher to their likely benefactors, the diet and drug industries.[34] Campos refers to several studies that follow this pattern: research from 1994 concluded that the majority of weight variance is genetic and unchangeable and as such, that most dieters will gain and lose weight cyclically, and weight cycling increases mortality. The authors conclude from their own data that "Most of the obesity research community has deemed such data [on the risks of weight loss] compelling – but not enough to state that weight loss attempts by obese people are dangerous." The authors of the paper state that "Nowadays, it is not uncommon to hear "diets don't work." In fact, diets do work. It is prescriptions to diet that fail because patients usually do not follow them." In this case, as in many cases with research about fatness and its relationship to health, researchers interpret their data by concluding that if they're wrong, it must be the fat person's fault and their personal responsibility.[144] Most obesity research in 2004 when *The Obesity Myth* was published was privately funded; less than 1 percent of the federal budget for medical research went to studying "obesity," even amid a supposed pandemic panic. Twenty years later, funding for research on "obesity" remains in the hands of the private sector, which, given the rise of drugs like Ozempic and Wegovy, will likely continue the cycle of pulling the alarm, blaming the individual, and selling the solution.

Even though the commercials at the gym tell me that Ozempic is not a "weight loss drug" and that it is used to aid patients with diabetes, and that it's not marketed or approved for people under 18, the rise in use of semaglutide (brand names Ozempic and Wegovy) as an obesity drug is on the rise. Yet again, a promise of thinness and "treat obesity" comes in the form of a pharmaceutical – this time, a subcutaneous injection, which under the name Wegovy is used to treat obesity in children as young as 12 with FDA approval.[145] This approval comes on the heels of the change in guidelines from the American Academy for Pediatrics in January 2023, which recommends the standard "diet and exercise" as a means of weight loss for children, but encouraged and paved the way for weight loss drugs such as semaglutide as a "booster" if "traditional methods" like diet and exercise are insufficient.

The American medical establishment's most recent promise of thinness is so popular, in fact, that its Danish manufacturer Novo Nordisk has had to put a hold on advertising and shipments of the drug to the United States to prevent shortages.[145] Serious side effects, *of course*, are "less common," but can include pancreatitis, liver damage, and tachycardia; animal studies suggest that thyroid cancer is also a potential risk.[146] The possible negative physical and emotional effects of the drug are still tenuous for its teenage population, especially since their bodies are still growing. It seems that fear of fatness rules the narrative, however; some advocates for use of the drug claim that not using semaglutide is actually riskier for teens, since being fat *might* lead to "serious health conditions" and "premature death." In an NBC article which interviewed teens and families who have used the drug, stories suggest that now that they're thin they participate in extracurricular activities, feel more confident, and have a life beyond their wildest dreams.[147] The common pattern among efforts at weight regulation for young people is to scare them thin, and these new drugs are no exception.

In the classroom, conversations that ask "who is paying for the outcome of this science?" are important to present to students when considering the rise in the use of these weight loss drugs, because though they are for use in people with diabetes and insulin resistance, they are increasingly being used as "quick fix" weight loss mechanisms and entering mainstream rhetoric. Secondary students are especially vulnerable to diet talk, the desire to lose weight to avoid social outcast, and may see hope and solutions in these drugs, which even the federal government is demanding more information about. Showing students the ways that science can be used to problematize their bodies can help them sift through information and make decisions about their health that are more comprehensively informed.

In a similar way that pharmaceutical companies and obesity research have become monetized, so has social media. Thus, the same question should frame students' conversations about what they see online, especially if it has claims that "science" is involved: Who is paying the creator of this content?

Weight loss drug advertising has even permeated professional sports broadcasting. In WNBA and college basketball, ads for companies like Ro and Hers, a purveyor of semaglutide drugs and other "wellness" products, are increasingly common. The Indiana Fever has an Eli Lilly patch deal on their jerseys.[148] When compared to sports assumed to be watched more frequently by men, such as NFL games, these ads are less frequent, but still there. Despite advertisers assuming that most football watchers are men (thus making weight loss ads less frequent than they may be between WNBA games), more than 50 percent of NFL fans are women[148] Hers and Hims spent more than $8 million to air a commercial targeting weight loss prescriptions and the weight-loss industry that "feeds on our failure."[149] The commercial, set to Childish Gambino's "This is America," claims that "obesity leads to half a million deaths each year."[150] Again, this is the same willful misinterpretation of correlation and causation, being used as fact despite being debunked in 1998. The commercial continues with "something's broken, and it's not our bodies; it's the system. There are medications that work; but they're priced for profits, not patients." The last 30 seconds of the minute long commercial touts their "affordable, doctor trusted" medications, a "treatment plan, designed by a doctor," and promises "you deserve to feel great in your body." How can you do that? By subscribing to their $199 monthly supply of weight loss drugs.[150]

The scary thing about ads like these is that they work. Studies have shown that 44 percent of watchers have visited a brand's website after seeing WNBA sponsorships during a game. Twenty-eight percent have bought from a sponsoring brand. Marketing research has also found that the three athletes who are most likely to convert consumers are Simone Biles, Serena Williams, and Angel Reese. And when young girls are watching, they are learning that there are quick fixes that can help them achieve a beauty standard like the ones they see on the court, side effects be damned. Girls aged 12–18 are the fastest-growing market for viewership of women's sports. This is "also the age group where they're going to be the most vulnerable for eating disorders."[148]

That's What Makes You Beautiful (Da Vinci Said So)

During the Renaissance, various artists competed for what they believed was the "ideal" measure of beauty and even sought to quantify it mathematically so they could represent it in their art. Leonardo Da Vinci was one such artist, and in addition to creating the Mona Lisa, he created what he called the "golden ratio" of the human form. The golden ratio is a mathematical equation applied to visual representations in art, with artists believing that the ratio of 1:1.618 makes "the most beautiful shapes." The ratio has also been called the golden proportion and the divine proportion, suggesting that beauty that falls into the realm of this exact geometrical calculation is in close proximity to a (Christian) higher power. The ratio is incorporated into various works like *The Wave of Kanagawa, the Last Supper, the Vitruvian Man*, and *the Mona Lisa* (Figure 5.1).[151]

Thus, the mission to represent human perfection was born. Of course, it's interesting that it was men, specifically mostly

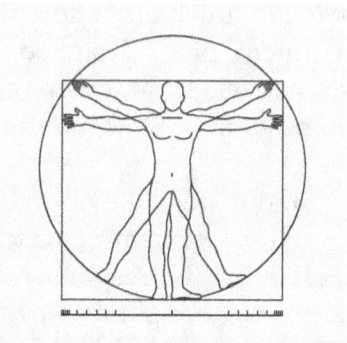

FIGURE 5.1 The "golden ratio" as demonstrated by Leonardo Da Vinci's "Vitruvian Man." Source: Shutterstock.

European men, studying women, most specifically European women, in search of what was true and unfiltered "beauty" … leaving out entire continents of people in the equation, just as Quetelet would do centuries later in search of *l'homme moyenne*. The construction of such a precise (and arbitrary) standard of beauty, of course when applied to people, suggests that anyone who doesn't meet it is "ugly," and therefore "inferior," or not close enough to God.[152] These same ideas born of Christian principles of spiritual "fitness" were used to create ugly laws that discriminated against people with "disfigurements," including "obesity." Fast forward to today, and there are "beauty scanner" apps that people can use to "measure" how their facial features add up to the golden ratio, or don't. These standards of beauty almost always did not apply to people of the global south either, which points to the attempt to quantify fair-skinned, thin, European bodies and faces as "the right way" to look.

Illustrator Mel Stringer credits paintings like those of Paul Gaugin, artists like Sophie Campbell and Yoshimoto Nara with her own journey finding herself and her body size represented in art. This shift led her to create art of her own that represents the same body type she grew up in, but didn't grow up seeing.[32]

Being fat hasn't always been aesthetically popular, but art reminds us that it was, in some societies, a testament to the human body's evolutionary power. Take, for example, ancient representations like the Venus of Willendorf, whose stoutness

Quick Tip

When showing and teaching about different art forms, styles, and standards of beauty, how can you include larger bodies – and discuss how they are represented across cultures, time periods, and visual imagery?

suggests that the fat body was idolized, especially during a time when life expectancy was low and food scarcity was high.[27] The common discourse surrounding representations of fatness in art often have to do with class (the fatter you were, the more access you had to food), but it also may point us to a more scientific discovery: that when the body isn't totally sure where it's next meal will come from, it holds onto fat to help the body survive. It's true that those who could afford paintings of themselves were also probably well-fed; but for everyday subjects in everyday life, the other possibility of fatness was the body's way of protecting itself from famine. Through this lens, the cultural possibility that anyone, of any social rank, could be fat, disrupts the idea that fatness was reserved for the rich in the way that today it is largely associated with the poor. After all, said Nina Simone, "it is an artist's duty to reflect the times."[153] Art can tell us a lot about what we value as a society, and body image (thinness) remains one of those values.

The visibility of size diversity shows students that bodies of all sizes are capable of creating, moving, and shaking the boundaries of our culture, and challenges the ideas of "beauty" that evolve as humans do. It also invites conversation about the ways that fat creators are hidden or not given credit for their work, and the ways that artists can ensure that their work remains theirs. Avoiding plagiarism is a lecture we give students all the time in the areas of research and content generation, and showing them examples of where our culture has fallen short on these ethical guidelines (and the ways that that shortcoming has often had implications of intersectional inequity) is a step in using creativity and criticality to push back against anti-fatness and other forms of bias.

Willie Mae "Big Mama" Thornton topped the charts. Thornton, who was born in Alabama in 1926, was most famous for her original song "Hound Dog," which is largely credited to Elvis Presley. Despite her success with the song, which spent 14 weeks on R&B hit charts, including seven weeks as number one on the 1953 *Billboard*, she saw only one royalty check for $500.[154, 155] Thornton's version of "Hound Dog" sold over 500,000 copies. Elvis, who heard a rendition of the song at a Las Vegas hotel, recorded it shortly after, never giving Big Mama credit. She died of a heart attack and liver disorders in a boarding house in Los Angeles, and was buried in a shared potter's field grave.[157]

> **Quick Tip**
>
> *Visual media is a valuable tool for asking students these questions:*
> *What or who is present in this story? What or who is missing from this story? What action must we take as readers, writers, and learners to ensure that missing voices are heard?*

One of the most surprising rabbit holes I ever fell down was learning the voice behind one of the most iconic songs of the 90s was a fat woman named Martha Elaine Wash. Known for her distinct belting of the lyric "Everybody dance now!," Wash was originally part of a female R&B duo called Two Tons O' Fun (a nod to both singers' larger figures) with Izora Armistead.[156] In the music video for the song "Gonna Make You Sweat (Everybody Dance Now)" by C + C Music Factory in 1990, the words are lip synced by Zelma Davis, a thin Black woman clad in a skin-tight black dress.[157] The song peaked at number one on the *Billboard Hot 100*, and Wash went uncredited for the vocals. Wash later filed a lawsuit against the group, prompting Sony to make a never-before-achieved request to MTV to add a disclaimer to the music video when it aired on their channel, crediting Wash with the vocals. The implication that Wash could not be the voice of the song, despite its iconic and powerful vocal range, because she is a fat woman, remains a product of anti-fat bias. In 2023, *Rolling Stone* magazine ranked Wash at number 179 on its list of the 200 Greatest Singers of All Time.[156]

Since her catapult to fame, Lizzo has maintained an on-and-off digital presence in the face of backlash, hate, and outright bigotry. As with any public figure, the visibility of celebrities is impossible to miss or avoid. Following Lizzo and reading her comments is not only a masterclass in self-love and shirking the confinement of beauty standards despite the haters, but a lesson in how our society sees fat people and thinks they can treat them from across a pixelated screen. As a cultural icon, Lizzo flies in the face of all the standards created by the men of centuries past. She is fat, Black, and unapologetic about both – and has risen to the top of media stardom for this bold statement of the fact of her existence.

Something that we often do when framing our discourse around cultural figures like Lizzo is hold them to a standard of respectability politics that ensures their survival and relevance. In exchange for performing the "good fat person" story we all believe is required to remain in the good graces of diet culture, Lizzo retains her relevance and popularity, even as people laugh at, not with, her for her size. Lizzo has to go "See? I work out/eat healthy/do cardio in the name of health" for us to see her as human. Lizzo has received criticism from virtually every corner of our culture for, most often, the crime of existing while fat, which many call "glorifying obesity," including celebrity fitness queen Jillian Michaels. The tune of this criticism falls flat, however, every time someone remembers that Lizzo is an artist; and that her entire career rests on her talent as a trained flutist and singer with multi-octave vocal range who does intense choreography during performances. Still, she has had to take several social media breaks for her mental health due to peoples' vitriol toward her appearance. Lizzo is not the only one whose self-worth is impacted by this cultural exchange. People in fat bodies – ones *without* millions of followers, platinum singles, and platforms – learn that in order to be seen as fully human, they must perform thinness and "health" to be offered access to humanity. Just look at the "funny fat friend" in any social group; among boys, he's often the football player who is fat "but he works out" and contributes to the culture of the team; in girls' social circles, the "funny fat girl" makes everyone laugh, even at her own expense. This paradigm is evidence that representation is not liberation – the presence of fat creators does not liberate us from fatphobia, especially if and when those creators subscribe to diet culture myths by performing the "good fat person" respectability that we require in order to accept them.

Our students have watched the bullying of a fat Black woman play out on social media a number of times, and some may participate in it themselves. Lizzo has made some grave missteps throughout her career; but the notable price she pays for being flawed while also being a woman, being fat, and being Black is unfairly wielded against her in the media with endless, often anonymous, aplomb. These three women in the music and creative art industries illustrate a well-crafted paradox of inequity: they are rendered invisible and hypervisible all at once.

Some contemporary fat lyricists I love whose messages can resonate with students are that of Mary Lambert and Kate Yeager. I cried to her original spoken word poem "Body Love" after discovering her through Macklemore & Ryan Lewis' LGBT ally anthem "Same Love" in 2014. She got me through the toughest of times with my body image and identity, and I've experienced the power of her musical talent firsthand. Mary Lambert also writes about fat, queer joy in songs like "Secrets," a pop song about being unapologetically fat, crying a lot, and living with bipolar disorder.

Kate Yeager, an artist based out of Nashville, wrote the song "Fat" (available on Spotify), which opens with a story about the first time someone ever called her fat – and how she learned that was supposed to be something she was ashamed of in that moment, changing the trajectory of her body image and self-esteem. Many of our students have this experience, and comparing them to artists who have similar messages of vague body positivity, like Jax's popular single "Victoria's Secret" can invite us to look at popular media and various artists' attempts to concentrate the narrative on body love instead of body shame.

> **Quick Tip**
>
> Craft a research project on their favorite songs and the creators behind them. What intersectionalities do they find in the production of their favorite art and music?

We...Totally Started the Fire

As the visual representation of culture, art is a powerful means of studying and understanding history. Anti-fat bias is one of many structures and systems we have not yet dismantled and continue to unlearn. Dr. Gholdy Muhammad, cited in Chapter

1, says that "we must name, understand, question and disrupt 'real-time' histories that are currently happening and problematic." Failing to recognize that anti-fat bias plays a role in other forms of oppression like racism, ableism, classism makes us, and our students, unable to do the work of unlearning the ways these constructions have taken up space in our consciousness. There are so many examples of policies, people, and practices that can illuminate the role of size diversity (and lack thereof) in history.

The aforementioned Venus of Willendorf statue, standing 4.4 inches tall, was an early Paleolithic representation of the fat female body that gave us clues about what size and shape was like 30,000 years ago.[158] The figurine was discovered during an excavation in 1908, a century after the real-life existence of Sara Baartman, a real life "Venus," from the Khoikhoi of the Eastern Cape province of South Africa.

Throughout Sara's life, her captors objectified her in "freak shows" around Europe after working as a maid, a wet nurse, and a washerwoman for Dutch and British families around South Africa. Her story is the story of lifelong exploitation, commodification, and violence, directly linked to her size. She was brought to London in 1810, and exhibited for her steatopygia – large amounts of tissue around the hips, butt, and thighs.[16, 159] Her figure was thought to be of scientific, medical, and erotic interest, and made her captors, Hendrik Cesars and Alexander Dunlop, large sums of money. Later in her life, she was sold to an animal trainer in France, who evaded slavery laws and displayed her as an exhibit at wealthy people's parties and private salons until he was deported.[16] After her death, her body was dismembered and parts of it were preserved for scientific inquiry.[16]

It is important to learn Sara Baartman's history because it ties together so much of what we've talked about in the content areas of science, health, beauty, art, and race and gender violence. All of these things cannot be separated from size discrimination, and our students see these histories repeat themselves in their social media content, books, TV, and movies, and their everyday lives. But teaching the history of how we view fat and people in larger bodies isn't just because we need to uncover more "hidden figures" and note their accomplishments – remember, representation alone is not liberation. Focusing our energy on the ways that inequity has happened because of size discrimination, and how it has led to movements focused on liberation and equity prioritizes an end to harm. As most of us know, we must learn from our history; lest we repeat it.

"Ugly Laws" in the 19th century in the United States ran parallel to the cultural pervasiveness of circus side shows. Such statutes were popping up all over America because of the eugenics movement. Ugly laws applied to people with physical disfigurements, disabilities, and even "obesity," to keep them from begging in the street because they were also often poor and destitute. The very first such law in the United States was created on July 9, 1867, in San Francisco. In addition to outlawing "street begging," the statute also stated that "any person who is diseased, maimed, mutilated, or in any way deformed so as to be an unsightly or disgusting object, or an improper person [...] shall not therein or thereon expose himself or herself to public view," laws passed in cities like Reno, Nevada, New Orleans, Chicago, Portland, Oregon were often positioned next to ordinances about racial integration, immigration, and vagrancy (loitering), thus positioning them firmly in our national effort to maintain a social hierarchy and eugenics.[160, 161] "Ugly" became synonymous with "socially unfit," and as the pseudoscientific efforts of people like Adolphe Quetelet, Louis Dublin, and others collided, fat people made their way into that category.

Such laws paved the way for employment discrimination based on appearance and disability, which would not be addressed until 1990 with the passage of the Americans with Disabilities Act (ADA). Even though being fat is not inherently disabling, the ADA was, and still is, the closest thing people in larger bodies had to defend themselves from employment discrimination based on their size. The lack of protection that fat people explicitly have before the law is a way that "ugly laws" silently persist.

As a result, fat people's job prospects and ability to exist in public left them few options for employment – thus their presence in "freak shows." Fat people's existence was relegated to public and self-objectification; and even in the face of this fascination, fatness remained both a subject and object of societal disgust.

In their article for *National Geographic*, author Ainsley Hawthorn states "Some justified the laws as a public health measure under the mistaken belief that seeing someone with a disability could literally make a healthy person sick."[160] This same argument is used to rally against the rise in fat-positive media representation, suggesting that even the sight of fat people in a neutral or positive way is "glorifying obesity" and will encourage people, especially young people, to "become fat." Another justification for ugly laws that echoes in today's understanding of fat bodies is the belief that "if disabled people were moved from the streets into institutions, they would receive better care." Institutionalizing and surveilling fat bodies is a way that we tell the people who live in them that there are systems that know them better than they know themselves, and that they are a "problem" to be regulated. What this actually does, in both cases, is "stripping disabled [and fat] individuals of their right to self-determination and isolating them from the rest of society." What ugly laws told us about fat people was that, according to nothing but cultural prejudice, fat people were too disgusting and unsightly to be seen in public and in everyday life; and this prejudice became the basis for medical "fact."

"Freak shows" added to the negative sensationalism of fat bodies in American and larger Western culture. Even before the health and medical professions decided that being fat was unhealthy, they believed it was grotesque, exotic, and bizarre. The freak shows of Europe, which featured women like Sara Baartman, were brought to the United States and popularized by P.T. Barnum.[162] Samuel Gumpertz, another circus pioneer, brought the freak show to Coney Island, which included short people, people with missing limbs, and fat people.[163] Since then, it has become the more body positive home of the "mermaid parade," an event that takes place during pride month to celebrate queer, and often, fat and Black bodies (with lots of glitter).[164]

Beyond the Victorian era, freak shows lasted through the Great Depression, when people all over America were hard-pressed for cash and could make a living in the circus. "Many a fat person, tired of being gawked at for free, joined the circus and was paid well to be the source of visual amusement."[163] One of the most famous examples is Ruth Smith, an Indiana native who weighed sixteen pounds at birth and 815 at the height of her fame. She performed for nearly ten years for the Ringling Brothers, Barnum & Bailey circus. Working-class Americans sometimes made themselves fat in order to join the circus, especially those who did not have much formal education and performed "unskilled" labor – in order to escape the financial woes of the Great Depression.[163] Middle-class Americans, who could not resist the curiosity of seeing her largeness for themselves, purchased tickets to sideshows that garnered her $400 a day; 4,000 in today's dollar value.[163] She died in 1942 at age 37 from weight loss surgery complications.

Though the American elite was somewhat shielded from the ways that fatphobia impacted them (it's easy not to care about others' opinion of you if you have the wealth, status, and privilege of tuning it out), public figures like William Howard Taft and William M. "Boss" Tweed were often criticized on the basis of their fatness.

Taft, the 27th President of the United States, still remains the subject of legend related to his corpulence. Noted as the "heaviest president in American history," Taft apparently weighed 340 pounds, and there is a story about him getting stuck in a bathtub that remains firm in American lore. Nearly a century after his presidency and his death, we're still fascinated by the size of Teddy Roosevelt's successor: enough so to write articles about it in the *Washington Post* as recently as 2017 (Figure 5.2).[165, 166]

Political cartoons emphasized figures like Taft and their corpulence to mock them. Instead of just attacking Tweed's corruption or Taft's foreign policy decisions, American disapproval of their political dealings played out on their bodies. Thomas Nast, considered the father of American political cartoons, drew over 140 depictions of Tweed,[166] many of which caricatured his size as a way of critiquing his corruption over Tammany Hall in New York City.

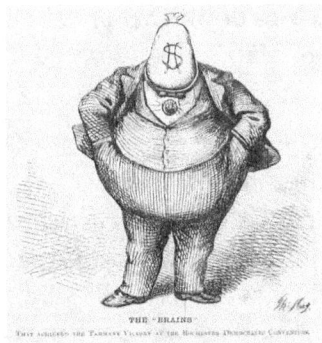

FIGURE 5.2 A well-known political cartoon by Thomas Nast depicting William "Boss" Tweed, published originally in Harper's Weekly in 1871. This image and others like it ushered in an era of normalizing the depiction of rich people as "fat cats," and associating greed and wealth with fatness.

Using fatphobia to make a political statement wasn't just exclusive to the United States. The Soviet Union often depicted capitalism by illustrating fat men in suits, surrounded by money, resembling pigs. The Nazis used similar imagery to illustrate Jewish people, whom they exclusively blamed for Germany's economic failure due to their widespread presence in jobs related to finance and banking – the only jobs they were allowed to have in many societies. On the contrary, the "ideal" German was blonde haired, blue eyed, and physically fit; ready to fight for the creation of a new Germany. In this case, anti-fat bias was often leveraged to propagandize war and genocide.

Quick Tip

When examining historical documents, especially imagery, invite students to think:

- *Why is the person, topic, or issue presented in this way? What is the goal of this image?*
- *Are there any credible or valid critical ideas we can discuss without talking about a person's body, size, or identity in a negative way?*

By 1940, the medicalization of disabilities often found in freak shows, and eventually also "obesity," led many to feel that there was "no place for freak shows in civilized society." Even Celesta Geyer, who replaced Ruth Smith in fat lady sideshow fame, went on to write a weight loss book *Diet or Die: Dolly Dimples' Weight Reducing Plan* in 1968, after suffering a near-fatal heart attack at 50 and reducing her weight from 555 to 112 pounds.[167]

What Fat Activists Can Teach Us

As the struggle for civil rights was underway in the 20th century, Americans in larger bodies sought for the laws to meet their bodies where they were as well. While people like Celesta Geyer changed their bodies amid rising anti-fat bias, others sought change and liberation from the bias itself. Activists like Steve Post founded NAAFA, the National Association to Aid Fat Americans, in July 1969, and their organizing stood adjacent to the fight for LGBTQIA+ and disability rights.[168] Inspired by Black activists who hosted sit-ins at lunch counters, such organizations came together to host a "fat in" where they ate publicly, chanted, carried signs, and burned diet books in Central Park.[168] This was the first mainstream presence of fat acceptance in America. Post's approach to fat liberation was largely through the male gaze, and gave way to creating spaces for fat people, and those who wanted to date them, space to socialize. Taking a more feminist approach that centered on liberation, human dignity, and body autonomy, two women set out on their own path to create a framework for fat activism – which became known as the Fat Underground. The two founders largely cultivated their ethos in a liberation network known as the Radical Therapy movement.[169] They, and other supporters of the movement, believed that mental illness was a function of larger scopes of oppression including racism, ableism, and fatphobia – and sought to change the paradigm for all people. She founded the Fat Underground with Sara Golda Bracha Fishman in Los Angeles, and it later folded into the L.A. NAAFA chapter.[170] Today, NAAFA has restructured and renamed to the National Association to Advance Fat Acceptance. Activists Judy Freespirit and Aldebaran set out from Los Angeles to split off from NAAFA to form the Fat Underground in 1972.[171, 172, 169] Critiquing the medical establishment's conceptions of what causes people to be fat, as well as applying radical liberatory radical therapy frameworks, intersectionality, and feminist theory, Fat Underground sought to

FAT   LIBERATION
MANIFESTO

1. WE believe that fat people are fully entitled to human respect and recognition.

2. WE are angry at mistreatment by commercial and sexist interests. These have exploited our bodies as objects of ridicule, thereby creating an immensely profitable market selling the false promise of avoidance of, or relief from, that ridicule.

3. WE see our struggle as allied with the struggles of other oppreressed groups against classism, racism, sexism, ageism, financial exploitation, imperialism and the like.

4. WE demand equal rights for fat people in all aspects of life, as promised in the Constitution of the United States. We demand equal access to goods and services in the public domain, and an end to discrimination against us in the areas of employment, education, public facilities and health services.

5. WE single out as our special enemies the so-called "reducing" industries. These include diet clubs, reducing salons, fat farms, diet doctors, diet books, diet foods and food supplements, surgical procedures, appetite suppressants, drugs and gadgetry such as wraps and "reducing machines".

   WE demand that they take responsibility for their false claims, acknowledge that their products are harmful to the public health, and publish long-term studies proving any statistical efficacy of their products. We make this demand knowing that over 99% of all weight loss programs, when evaluated over a five-year period, fail utterly, and also knowing the extreme proven harmfulness of frequent large changes in weight.

6. WE repudiate the mystified "science" which falsely claims that we are unfit. It has both caused and upheld discrimination against us, in collusion with the financial interests of insurance companies, the fashion and garment industries, reducing industries, the food and drug industries, and the medical and psychiatric establishment.

7. WE refuse to be subjugated to the interests of our enemies. We fully intend to reclaim power over our bodies and our lives. We commit ourselves to pursue these goals together.

FAT PEOPLE OF THE WORLD, UNITE! YOU HAVE NOTHING TO LOSE ....

By Judy Freespirit and Aldebaran
November, 1973

Published by the Fat Underground, P. ████████████████

FIGURE 5.3 From the Fat Liberation Archives, fatlibarchive.org.

be a liberatory space for fat Americans, especially those with multiple marginalities (Figure 5.3).[172, 168]

While Fat Underground dissipated by 1983, NAAFA remains intact with 11,000+ members as of this writing. Critics of NAAFA, and of fat acceptance in general, say that NAAFA "is an apologist for an unhealthy lifestyle. But NAAFA says it does no such thing, that some people are just bigger and no less deserving of the same rights as everyone else."[168] NAAFA remains critical of the weight loss industry and weight loss surgery in particular, because of its complications and the stigma delivered to fat people by both. Today, all the materials gathered, published, and created by the Fat Underground exist in the Fat Liberation Archive, which contains zines, flyers, leaflets, articles, and photos dated by decade starting in the 1960s.

Fat activists offer many lessons historically, including the history of how achieving status in society has often been about being in the "right" body and how marginality, oppression, and liberation play out on our physical selves. The ultimate message that "the personal is political" happens in and on fat bodies and spaces, and fat activists have, in many cases, been in several different fights for human and civil rights at once – especially during the 20th century.

I don't list any "first" fat people to do whatever in this section because teaching history is about more than tokenizing the first people to do something or celebrating one singular person who broke barriers. What that does is effectively mythologizes the struggle of being fat, Black, indigenous, queer, disabled, an immigrant, and marginalized – representation is important, but even more important is solidarity and the creation of an equitable future so that there don't have to be more aspirational, inspirational "firsts" we make movies out of and fawn over – existing in a world where equity is the norm is how history is really made. People who were the first are really important, but more important is, how did they prop the door open for the people behind them, and make sure they could fit through it? Stories of people who made it out (with or without intersecting privileges) will not liberate us on their own. Questioning and changing policy and demanding better, like so many of the people I admire did, will build us new worlds.

Talk to Me

Since the WHO has globalized the "obesity epidemic," world language classes have taken on the topic as a means of discussing cultures around the world. The WHO operates on a model of "western" (white) medicine, with little room for indigenous ways of being and respect for cultural differences. Even the word "obesity" and its origins are fraught with the implication of personal responsibility; the word comes from the Latin "obesus" meaning "having eaten until fat," and obesitas, or "to be very fat." The WHO has made it plain that "obesity" as a condition is entirely "preventable."[173] This is evident in their alarmism around the globalization of "obesity," and fails to acknowledge that there are fat people everywhere in the world, and they are fat for a number of reasons – and none of those reasons deserve to be pathologized, monitored or corrected.[174] Here's what the WHO says about obesity:

> Paradoxically coexisting with undernutrition, an escalating global epidemic of overweight and obesity – "globesity" – is taking over many parts of the world. If immediate action is not taken, millions will suffer from an array of serious health disorders.

> Obesity is a complex condition, one with serious social and psychological dimensions, that affects virtually all age and socioeconomic groups and threatens to overwhelm both developed and developing countries. In 1995, there were an estimated 200 million obese adults worldwide and another 18 million under-five children classified as overweight. As of 2000, the number of obese adults has increased to over 300 million. Contrary to conventional wisdom, the obesity epidemic is not restricted to industrialized societies; in developing countries, it is estimated that over 115 million people suffer from obesity-related problems.[174]

I have seen lessons on "obesity" in Italy and other countries, and unsurprisingly, in these lessons the same pictures we use in America to talk about fat people – photos of bodies without heads and hands consuming burgers and fries. Such lessons illustrate the ways that fear of fat is culturally pervasive, and spreading worldwide. In an ENL lesson developed by a teacher in England,[175] available on their personal site for $9.99, one of the tasks asks students to rank different foods like "fries, chocolate, cheesecake, pizza, kebabs, burgers, potato chips and steak" by which is the "worst," putting the "worst" food at the top. It does not define what "worst" means, which is an arbitrary way of moralizing food. Other activities packaged in the lesson include word studies of articles about the global obesity epidemic from BBC, *The Guardian*, and *The Hill*, including words like gloomy, obese, abnormal, excessive, and adolescent; all of which in this context are presumed to have negative connotations.[174]

In a lesson for English language learners, the consideration that some of the foods on this list – kebabs, for instance, which originated in Turkey and are commonly eaten throughout the Mediterranean and the Middle East – might be a student's cultural food, which the teacher contextualizes on a list of foods that are the "worst." The list is also entirely subjective, and does not discuss the nutritional value in each – despite there being adequate sources of protein, vegetables, grains, dairy, and more on the list. Another activity in the lesson plan asks students to discuss questions like "How many people will be obese by 2035?" and "What might there be in the future if we don't act now?"[76] The line of questioning here is rooted in a sense of urgency and paternalism, and problematizes fat bodies just for existing; it is culturally problematic and casts understanding of food, culture, and bodies in the western gaze.[177]

Another lesson titled "la Obesidad in Mexico," created for an intermediate Spanish class, presents questions like "What are the dangers of obesity? Which populations are at risk for being overweight or obese?" The lesson plan, which is available for purchase for $18.99, uses the "problem" of "obesity" in Mexico to teach skills like present tense regular verbs, present tense irregular verbs, noun-adjective agreement, and cognates.[178] The authors of the lesson are two white teachers from Ohio, pointing again to the positioning of bodies of color, in this case Mexicans, as "wrong," in need of regulation and monitoring, and whose cultural practices presumably "cause" their fatness. The lesson, however, is billed as "comparing cultural perspectives," but does not seem to be written by anyone who is part of the culture that the lesson is examining.

Justice for Piggy

Stories connect us as humans – it's why I was drawn to the content area when I became an educator. Narrative is an art that asks us to find empathy in our lived experience and shared humanity. The push to read, write, and talk about stories that make students feel represented and let them know their identities matter is one that has not fully extended to fat students and their lives, however.

One of the things I love most about teaching ELA is presenting students with new ways of looking at language. "Fat" has become a word we've culturally internalized as an insult, and hurled it across playgrounds and even online spaces. We've been socialized to use specific language about size, and internalize what use of that language means about bodies and their worth.[11] This part is where being a teacher of the English language and its function comes in handy: because in the realm of my content area, there's a word for the negative charge we've given to fat – connotation. And when we can teach that connotation, unpack its origins, and disarm the weight of the hatred levied against the people who embody that adjective, we can see fat bodies and size diversity as a fact of our human existence. In her essay for Angie Manfredi's anthology *The Other F Word: A Celebration of the Fat and Fierce* (a text I highly recommend placing in the high school ELA classroom), author Jes Baker says that for her, "the word fat is not inherently bad. It's a simple adjective. It's a neutral descriptor of the size of my body."[32]

She says,

> "This word, while something that I'm happy to use, still makes many others deeply uncomfortable. Their discomfort often causes them to jump to my 'defense' ..." You're *insert every other socially preferred euphemism here*." We will call ourselves and fat people "chubby, fluffy, curvy," and "plus-sized" before we ever utter the word fat, and that comes with not wanting to offend anyone – but it also comes from a deep-seated fear of becoming what we have

been told the word fat means – lazy, slovenly, sluggish, gluttonous, undisciplined, disgusting, the list goes on. Baker says that "It's the dots we connect between the word and someone's worth that is harmful, and THAT is the part we must change."[32]

Whenever I think about the fat characters and storylines that do exist in books, I think of characters like Piggy from *Lord of the Flies*, who, of course, is depicted as so annoying that he is the first to be killed in the text. Characters like Piggy are disposable; comic relief; the sidekick; and a host of other tropes that reduce fat bodies to the background (unless, of course, they pull off a weight loss "redemption arc"). In the same way we can reposition inherently neutral words like "fat" into being just descriptors, we must unpack the use of animals to talk about fat people. What does it really mean when we call someone a "whale," an "elephant" or a "pig"? What are we saying about how we see their humanity in relation to their size?

This highlights that it isn't enough to have fat characters *exist* in books; the representation of them and their experiences must reflect full lives that don't require them to change anything before they get the guy or girl, save the day, or win the prize. What we teach students when we don't push back at narratives that dehumanize fat bodies, in any genre, is that those bodies somehow earned our dislike, our disdain, or in Piggy's case, their demise.

"To incorporate stories that feel real and like they're talking about important issues like anti-fat bias, but that don't feel like an after school special is crucial," says Crystal Maldonado, author of *Fat Chance, Charlie Vega,* and other books with fat protagonists. Stories like the ones she describes show students that there is no weight limit to success; and that success doesn't have to equal weight loss, either.

Again, the adage "representation isn't complete liberation" bears repeating. Including texts with fat characters in them is a pivotal step in creating inclusion of all bodies, but what is being said about those bodies? Do they reinforce diet and weight loss narratives as part of the story? Are they available as independent reading options, or whole class novels to study widely and deeply together for further inquiry? Building a robust, diverse, and representative classroom library is important in making students feel seen and heard and for introducing students to experiences that aren't their own. This is how empathy grows. But when we reduce all the "diverse books" to classroom library reads, we show students that these voices are optional to learn about. What would it look like to read a book like *Charlie Vega* or *Starfish* as a whole class, and talk about the issues of fatphobia and weight stigma as you notice them together?

> Incorporating these stories would help with dealing with diet culture and anti-fat bias, with helping students see how the world is not set up in a way that's not set up equitable for everyone; everyone has different experiences and how do we talk about experiences with understanding and care?

Crystal said. It's hard to frame conversations about students who may be in the room, who may have internalized that their bodies are the problem; but she says,

> Books can make important topics not feel so pointed – it's hard to open up as a young person, but when there's a character in a fictional story it makes it so much easier to point out the bias and their own experiences of discrimination.

If they are reading about characters like Charlie Vega, who is a reflection of Crystal's own experience, or Ellie from Lisa Fipps' *Starfish*, or Willowdean in Julie Murphy's *Dumplin'*, it allows the kids who these stories feel like they're about to see that they're not alone for a number of reasons: (1) a fictional character has been created that is living some of what they know to be true and (2) if the text is an own-voices text, that usually means that the author, a real person, has been through it, too.

> Charlie Vega is the closest to my life and my life experience – that battle between wanting to love yourself

and accept yourself for who you really are, but having to trudge through all these feelings she's getting from society, from her own mom – so many of us in fat positivity and body positivity deal with that in real life. I absolutely would go to bat for anyone and talk about how all bodies are good bodies and fat folks deserve justice, but there's still this feeling that we're different and that maybe that means we're not worthy of good things,

she shared.

The existence of bad representation does not mean that bad representation isn't valuable, though. Many classic texts, which are required by the curriculum across states and in international programs, offer poor, negative, or stereotypical representations of fat people and their experiences. These texts are opportunities to unpack our own cultural mistreatment of real fat people, and divorce our thinking about them from the stereotypes we've all learned. If you are in a school where the curriculum requires you to teach the classics, spend time reading the text carefully and critically for fat characters. How are they represented? What words are used to describe them? How might you present this to students, or ask them to think about it? Critical lenses are an important part of studying literature, and fat studies is one we can add to our repertoire among the ones we ask students to notice: race, class, gender, power, and so on. One such example is in William Golding's *Lord of the Flies*; starting with his name, he is nicknamed after an animal, and not just any animal – one noted for its size, stubbornness, filth, and slovenliness. Piggy, perhaps the most intelligent of all the boys, is seen as annoying, called anti-fat names, and constantly derided by their leader, Jack. He is eventually brutally killed, signaling his disposability as a character and perhaps revealing the author's own attitudes toward people like him, to boot.

Debbie Saroufim, a Los Angeles-based body image coach, talked with me about her approach to literature discussion with her own kids: "I love the *Harry Potter* series because it offers so much," she says. "I don't love the author, but I love the conversations that books like these can help us have." Saroufim refers to the author's continued (and very public) transphobia and overt fatphobia that show up in her writing, but invites even her own kids to critically push back against the narratives presented by such biases. One such example she offers is the presentation of Dudley, Harry's cousin who is always framed as being mean, rude, and unkind to Harry alongside descriptions of his fat body. "We can talk about the ways that Dudley is just not a very nice cousin, in ways that have nothing to do with his body," she said. Teaching texts from this critical framework allows us to see characters for their dimensions, good and bad; and unravel the cognitive association we have with size and poor character.

Teaching texts that show students the full range of fat experience is one way that weight stigma can meet its overdue demise in the ELA classroom. One of my favorite authors to teach in a whole-class setting is the poet Rachel Wiley and her work. She writes about a variety of topics, namely about being fat, queer, biracial, and a woman. Her poem "The Fat Joke" is one I've taught from grades 8 to 12, and it is an invitation to my students to see a fat person who is not interested in shrinking themselves – who instead calls out fatphobia, even from her doctor. My students have reacted in a number of ways to her work over the years, but one thing that it affords them is that seeing people in larger bodies is not optional. We confront the paradox of seeing fat bodies because of their bigness, and the ways that society renders them subhuman, invisible, and unworthy.

The visibility of fat authors, characters, and narratives is equally as important as fat joy. It is not enough to represent fat characters, fat authors, and fat people – but helping students understand and recognize that larger bodies can and do experience joy, love, hope, laughter, desirability, and the mundane help us combat the narrative that they are unlovable, lazy, not smart, not motivated, and that their fatness is the worst thing that could possibly happen to them.

Big Moves for ELA Teachers

Nonfiction

♦   *Body Talk: 37 Voices Explore our Radical Anatomy* edited by Kelly Jensen
♦   *The Other F Word: Stories of the Fat and Fierce* edited by Angie Manfredi

Fiction

♦   *Fat Chance, Charlie Vega* by Crystal Maldonado
♦   *Big Fat Manifesto* by Susan Vaught
♦   *Starfish* by Lisa Fipps
♦   *Dumplin'* by Julie Murphy
♦   *Camp Sylvania* by Julie Murphy
♦   *Fat Angie* by E.E. Charlton-Trujillo

Poetry

♦   *Fat Girl Finishing School* by Rachel Wiley
♦   "Song of Myself" by Walt Whitman
♦   *Song of My Softening* by Omotara James

Mind Your Media

The lack of size diversity, or limited narratives of fat characters in fiction as having only negative traits, comes from our real-life presentations and ideas of *people* in fat bodies. Conversations around body acceptance and weight stigma in the classroom must ensure that fat bodies aren't up for debate. In my own classroom practice, we host an argument unit that includes a spoken debate. As a rule, debating people's humanity or inherent dignity is off the table. Questions like "Should we ban immigration?" or "Should LGBTQ+ people be allowed to marry?" are debate questions that hang people's equal access to participation in our society in the balance. The right of people in larger bodies to access our society is no different. Questions like "Should we ban junk food at school?" strengthen the narrative that there are "good" and "bad" foods, and throw a sideways glance at the students who eat them. We should avoid topics like this as much as possible.[179]

That doesn't mean that students can't debate about the *policies* created about their bodies at school. In Chapter 6, we'll talk about the school cafeteria, and there is much to be debated about the ways that media and product research play out in our schools – with kids as the target consumers.

Big Moves for Debate

♦ Should companies be allowed to advertise their products in schools?
♦ Should we learn more about what kinds of food are served at school, and where it comes from?
♦ Does our school source our cafeteria food from ethical sources?
♦ Should our school be able to ban certain foods and food groups from being sold in our cafeteria?
♦ Does our school dress code discriminate against certain people's bodies and not others?
♦ Should recess be required for all schools in the United States.?
♦ What does our school do to prevent or cut down on food waste?
♦ Does our school do enough to address bullying that happens to people about their size or weight?
♦ Propose a change to one school policy that you believe is harmful to students' body image or self-esteem.

Though at this point older than students in our classrooms, *Shallow Hal* (2001) is available on Disney+ alongside movies and series our students know, love, and watch regularly. This film, starring Gwenyth Paltrow and Jack Black, is supposed to be a romantic comedy about a man who, after being hypnotized into only being able to see a person's inner beauty, falls in love with a woman (played by Gwenyth Paltrow in a fat suit) who he believes to be beautiful (thin) but is really 300 pounds; a trait the audience is supposed to equivocate with ugliness. The delusion of Hal, the main character, as to her true form is supposed to be the punchline of the whole film. But beyond that, we are supposed to believe that what's funny about *Shallow Hal* is that fat people could not possibly be lovable, desirable, or even possible partners.[34]

When images like these become part of our consciousness, they become part of who we believe fat people *are*. These same ideas, coupled with thousands of articles about an "obesity epidemic" that was created over the course of decades by various industries, are a recipe for bias; making media literacy about body image and anti-fatness critical across grade levels.

The film was nominated in several categories at the 2002 Teen Choice Awards[180] – which is alarming, considering the implication that this means that the film, which punches down at women in larger bodies, was supposed to be funny and appropriate for a teen audience. Following the film, Gwenyth Paltrow revealed that being in a fat suit in public while filming was humiliating. She said,

> I almost cried, I was hurting so much inside. What I realized then, as well as from talking to overweight people, is that people think they are being kind by not looking, but that's the cruelest thing they can do. It makes the person feel so isolated.[34]

By her own admission, Paltrow was at least somewhat able to garner an understanding of what weight stigma does to marginalize and oppress others – and yet, over 20 years later, she built goop, a subscription-based empire of "wellness" products ranging from $27 underwear (on sale) to essential oils Gwenyth's $274 skincare routine.[181]

> Thin people, it seems, are finally beginning to hear what activists have been saying for decades: that our world is set up to be uniquely hostile to fat people at every possible turn, and that fat people are blamed for it.[182]

Celebrating body diversity and self-care with an asterisk (or a $200 price tag) is not celebration; it's gatekeeping and oppression. Moreover, Paltrow got to momentarily wear oppression as a costume that she could remove, and her only insight into the experiences that fat people endure every day in the medical industry, fashion industry, and workplace was "talking" to us.

More recent in our students' media consciousness is the rise of the Kardashian-Jenners. The women of this business, beauty, and media family have authored beauty standards as we know them. Alongside their reality TV series *Keeping Up with the Kardashians*, people worldwide have been able to keep up with Kris, Kim, Khloe, and Kourtney on social media. As they grew up, Kylie and Kendall entered the fray as well, following in their sisters' footsteps as trendsetters in beauty and lifestyle. The problem? Keeping up with the Kardashians is, quite literally, next to impossible (unless, of course, you have generational wealth).

And still, their reality TV show and their presence on social media offer modeling for parasocial relationship building in our culture. Parasocial relationships refer to "one-sided relationships in which a person develops a strong sense of connection, intimacy, or familiarity with someone they don't know." These relationships exist only in the mind of the individual, who experiences a bond despite the lack of reciprocity.[183] With celebrities like the Kardashians, Instagram, and Twitter allow us access to their lives, their content, and their messaging at virtually all times; and the mark they've left on the consciousness of viewers now reaches beyond them. Such views of public figures allow us to feel like we really know them, and take the idea of "role model" a step too far. Social media has offered us access to celebrity figures like Kim Kardashian, and that constant (one-sided) contact gives us an opportunity not only to wish we could be like them, but also we could *be* them.

Nearly all the women in this family have been criticized publicly for filtering their social media photos, promoting diet products like "flat tummy shakes" and crash dieting to fit into designer clothes for public appearance events.[184] Like Gwenyth Paltrow, they have admitted to struggling with body image and hinted at acknowledging that the way they look is unrealistic, if not achieved by surgical and chemical means; but still, they build brands on selling the dream of changing your body to fit their mold to the world. Kim's body image has been the stuff of studies on its impact on women and girls. A study done for York University in Toronto found that for consumers of Kardashian-related media, the constant posts of "slim thick" body types are bad for body image. The 400 research participants aged 18–25 viewed 13 photos of "slim thick" influencers, and reacted to what they saw and how it made them feel.[105] The study actually named the Kardashian mogul and her sister Kylie Jenner as influencers who contribute to the discontent women feel about their bodies because of their online content. The "slim-thick" body ideal, which features a smaller waist and flat stomach but larger breasts, butt, and thighs –has become increasingly popular in mainstream and social media in recent years.[185] The study found that such images actually had a worse effect on viewers' body dissatisfaction than photos of thin models. In 2016, after Kylie publicly admitted that she got lip filler, the American Society for Plastic Surgeons reported an increase in lip plastic surgery and related procedures.[186] Two years later, they did a study that procedures to modify the buttocks had increased by 256 percent since 2000 (despite being the most deadly cosmetic procedure)[187]; a likely side effect of Kim's cover photo for *Paper* magazine, featuring a photo of her opening a bottle of champagne that appears to be fizzing toward her protruded butt with the words "Break the Internet, Kim Kardashian" in white typeface at the bottom of her black leather dress.

It seems, though, that not even the Kardashians can keep up with the Kardashians. In an episode of their reality TV series, Kylie is shown breaking down over comments she's received online about looking "old," as a result of choosing to wear less makeup and dissolve her lip filler. Her twin sister, Kylie, has also said that it would "break her heart" if her daughter Stormi were to augment herself surgically the way she did as a young adult.[187, 188] Though the Jenner twins were more or less thrust into the spotlight unwillingly, they continue to have an impact on the body image and motivations of their followers. They [the media and the public] have been, she says, talking about her body and her body image since she was 12 and 13 years old.

Just one month after Kylie's tearful moment aired in June 2024, fitness influencers on TikTok were posting grueling workouts to achieve what they branded Kendall and Kylie's "yacht shoulders" – slim, chiseled shoulders accompanied by a thin neck and prominent collar bone.[188] This time, though, the sisters did not aim to set a trend; the Jenner girls were just existing in bathing suits, on a yacht in Mallorca. One post, of a woman nicknamed "PP" doing a workout to get these "yacht shoulders" reached 7.6 million viewers on the app. Such a phenomenon highlights the ways that some trends are connected to parasocial relationships. The Jenner girls weren't doing anything, didn't coin the term themselves – but looking like them became a body ideal.

In addition to giving the world 24/7 access to the Kardashian-Jenner family to compare ourselves to, social media is to thank for what we've come to know as the "body positivity" movement. Body positivity, however, has become fraught with problems; including the centering of the most normative bodies – thus, defeating the purpose of the movement at all. Body positivity, it seems, comes with certain limitations; there are rules for how one can express love for themselves, and just how much a person is allowed to love themselves before they are accused of "glorifying obesity."

Related to the aspiration toward "yacht shoulders" is the pervasive online-gone-IRL insult "big back." Topping over 174 million posts on TikTok, the trendy phrase is the latest in fat-shaming lingo. The trend involves recording yourself or someone else eating a lot or stuffing your clothes to make your back appear bigger than it is. The trend makes a spectacle out of eating, and associates any and all eating with "fatty" behavior – creating insecurity around food consumption and making a mockery of fat people.[189] "That tends to reinforce this idea that if you're in a bigger body, you're always consuming massive amounts of food. It reinforces that notion of gluttony," said Oona Hanson in an article for *Fortune* magazine.[189]

The harm of terms like "big back" are many, but the most significant is that it creates anxiety around eating in public, especially because it is commonly a joke among thin kids. Eating is a normal physical and social behavior, and shaming that behavior, whether or not it resembles binging, is a surefire way to create hypervigilance and anxiety around food. Many teens interviewed in the same *Fortune* article said they would "never say it to an actual fat person," but remains as a joke among thin friends. The punchline serves the purpose of painting starvation in a positive light, suggesting that having the willpower and discipline not to respond to the call of simply eating a meal when hungry is a thing of virtue.

Chanea Bond, an ELA teacher in Texas is also quoted in the article, and says that in her experience, use of the phrase "started this school year. At first it was mostly students referring to themselves. But now 'big back' is so common in their vernacular, they say it anytime there's eating happening."[189]

Judging by teens' responses in the article, the knowledge that using this term as a trend in the way it has been stems from anti-fat stereotypes about fat bodies is there, but positions it so that they are off the hook for not acting out that harm against the people who would be hurt the most. This awareness does not make the use of terms like "big back" any better or more acceptable.

Quick Tip

Anytime harmful trends (especially those that originate online) come to your attention, make a plan to talk about them and ask students to think about them critically. With trends like "yacht shoulders" and "big back" as well as other body-focused phrases, ask questions like:

◆ Why do people find this kind of content funny or entertaining?
◆ Who might be harmed by this phrase/action/behavior?
◆ What can we do or say to disrupt these trends when we hear or see them? Why is that important?

Body positivity has become far removed from its intention of helping people love the skin they're in, and instead, is littered with images of "girls discussing their fitness journeys," weight loss advice, and trying to hide their features through filters. Many thin influencers contort themselves to show off bloated bellies and make themselves seem more "relatable," as if fatness is a costume.[190] "Now, just as in the past, constantly seeing images of supposedly ideal bodies can invite comparison and self-judgment, making young people feel worse about themselves," says Anna North, a *Vox* reporter. She cites a *Wall Street Journal* report that found that 32 percent of girls in a study about social media use said that "when they already felt bad about their bodies, Instagram made them feel worse." [191] North also mentions studies that found that among British teens, suicidal thoughts, pathological eating concerns, and depression were tied to adolescents' use of Instagram.[192]

Body positivity has also come up against the dangerous online presence of "pro ana" and "pro mia" accounts, which are users who promote behaviors like anorexia and bulimia. "Pro-eating disorder" content has been on social media and the Internet at-large since 2001, when Yahoo! deleted more than 113 pro-anorexia websites from its servers.[193]

Many creators of such content promote eating disorders not as an illness, but as a lifestyle choice; still other creators acknowledge the harm of the disorder they are experiencing and don't wish it for others, but post content that can trigger feelings of "thinspiration" nonetheless. Websites like Tumblr are credited with the creation of "thinspiration," which lives on on more popular platforms like Instagram, X (Twitter), Pinterest, and Snapchat.[194] Though the terms of use policies of many popular social media apps (which require users to certify that they are at least thirteen years old to use), big tech companies like Meta are under fire for their perceived failure to protect users from content that promotes eating disorders, especially among minors. Platforms like Instagram, Reddit, and TikTok have features that auto-detect certain search terms, like "anorexia," and direct users to resources like NEDA or 988, the newly fashioned U.S. suicide prevention hotline. In a 2021 U.S. Congressional hearing, Meta submitted internal research data that confirms that platforms like Instagram may be connected to declining adolescent mental health.[193, 194]

The anonymity provided by social media, coupled with herd mentality, may mean that bullying fat kids is more prevalent online.[69] Clark et al. argue that "The critical influence of social media in shaping beliefs may also lead to the internalization of weight stigma."[195] Samantha Lai, who wrote an article about social media's "eating disorder problem" for the Brookings Institution, suggests a solution to this problem:

Instead of simply linking to the NEDA webpage, social media companies should take a more proactive and involved approach. Theories on inoculation have shown that people become more resilient to political misinformation when they have been told to prepare for it. Similarly, social media companies could ensure that their users are better primed for harmful narratives surrounding diet culture and eating disorders by preemptively challenging harmful narratives. This could involve working with NEDA and other healthcare experts to create informational graphics, short videos, or easy-to-read Q&A resources.[196]

One survey they presented involved research from various countries and user ages. One such survey of 2,500 teens in the U.K. and United States reported that one in five teens says that Instagram makes them feel worse about themselves, though a small percentage (6–13 percent) of teens said that those feelings started on Instagram. While it may not be a *cause* of teens' body dissatisfaction, anxiety, and depression, it certainly isn't helping. One British teen who took the survey stated:

> You can't ever win on social media. If you're curvy, you're too busty. If you're skinny, you're too skinny. If you're bigger, you're too fat. But it's clear you need boobs, a booty, to be thin, to be pretty. It's endless, and you just end up feeling worthless and shitty about yourself.[195]

A prescription from across the pond offered by the Children's Hospital of Eastern Ontario Research Institute found that cutting a teen's scrolling time in half can "significantly" improve their body image in weeks.[195, 196]

Despite this public condemnation of promoting eating disorders in the media – social media, news media, and otherwise – Americans especially are subject to constant contradictions from various sources. Supersize your meal, but don't get fat. Lose weight, but don't starve yourself doing it. It's no wonder pharmaceutical companies are being looked to for solutions, even despite the risks we don't know about yet. Living in a culture of contradiction means it's hard for anyone, including teens and kids, to get conclusively accurate, helpful, or safe information about what to do with their bodies. [197]

Facilitating opportunities for students to spot the language of dieting and diet culture is also the work of media literacy. The diet has been rebranded to safeguard companies like Weight Watchers from the liability of promoting disordered eating, thinking, and exercise. Instead, what we know as a diet has been recast as a "lifestyle change," or even as "chronic restrained eating" in some cases.[34]

Denise Austin rose to acclaim as a spokeswoman for Reebok, advertising their first athletic shoe designed for women. Austin, who today emphasizes staying away from "crazy claims" of quick fixes and fad diets, once ran television programs titled *Get Fit and Lite* and *Denise Austin's Daily Workout*, which aired on ESPN2 before eventually moving to Lifetime.[198, 199] In 2001, she published a book that suggested a caloric intake of 1,500 calories per day, which, accompanied by her famous "fat burning" workouts, is a significant caloric deficit that even nutritionists consider a starvation diet. In the years since, she has said that she exercises just 30 minutes a day, does not skip meals, and prefers butter and sugar over artificial sweeteners.[34, 199] A year later, she was chosen by the Bush Administration to serve on the President's Council on Physical Fitness and Sports. Today at age 66, she says that she "walks because it brings her so much joy" and that she's been working out for 40 years, so there's "no excuse" why anyone can't do the same. The "no excuses" rhetoric reads as the jump from diet to lifestyle change; the suggestion that while dieting is bad, of course, there is a superior way to live (fit) that is attainable if we just stop letting life get in our way. There is so much potential for advocating for joyful movement here, and though advocating for natural means of achieving fitness is a positive one, is it overshadowed by the short distance that figures like Austin have helped pave from fitness and health to the desire to be thin?

Jillian Michaels, like Denise Austin, began her popularity streak as a fitness maven on social media and on television. Her show, *The Biggest Loser*, ran for 18 seasons on prime time television from 2004 to 2016, and was infamous for its scenes of Michaels screaming at and berating fat contestants whose mission was to lose (hopefully) significant amounts of weight under her watch.[200] The approach of bullying fat people into "shape" – literally – has become a source of not only modeling for how to treat fat people in real life, but morbid cultural entertainment. Contestants lost up to ten pounds per week while filming, with some losing up to 30 pounds in week one; a fact that goes against sound healthy reduction practices of one to two pounds per week. Losing this much weight this fast (especially through more than six hours per day of strenuous exercise that they do on the show) can weaken the heart muscle and lead to electrolyte and potassium deficits.[201, 202]

> **Quick Tip**
>
> *Ask students to write down a list of characteristics or behaviors they believe are "healthy" and ones that are "unhealthy." Ask them to explain their reasoning and the origin of that belief.*

Michaels' methods contradict the well-founded knowledge that weight cycling is worse for health than being fat and staying that way; and her subsequent endeavors, such as *30 Day Shred*, put forth the same cultural messages that the show does; that you can get fit and stay fit, as long as you keep buying what she's selling.

The show's methods have been questioned and even openly criticized by nutritional and health professionals, but that criticism feels a lot like striking a particularly juicy sentence that a lawyer knows will sway the jury: *The Biggest Loser*, whether we know it's harmful or not, has helped solidify negative perceptions of fat people and how to treat them in our society. The series serves as a modern-day "freak show," objectifying fat bodies for American entertainment and fascination. In the first phase of the show's formula, which begins with a challenge of temptation, tropes about fatness are presented as a fact of the contestants' lives, and framed as the reason they're there in the first place. They undergo a "challenge," which requires contestants to begin by eating high-calorie (but delicious) foods in exchange for things like calling their family, a mystery prize, or giving up workout time with that episode's trainer for a chance to win cash.[92] Considered a test of their willpower and willingness to be the "biggest loser," this challenge and its subtext suggest that all fat bodies became fat bodies by way of sugar, fat, and carbs – and that we'd choose those over money, exercise, or even our families.[203, 204, 205]

> **Quick Tip**
>
> *Using tools such as Harvard University's Implicit Bias test, invite students to challenge their perceptions of fat bodies and the people who occupy them; start with the media they consume on TV, social media apps, and in films. Remind students that implicit bias need not be a source of shame; given the pervasive nature of anti-fat messaging in the media, we are all susceptible to such ideas.*

The songs we sing to ourselves on repeat about fat people and their willpower become the ways our students treat fat people, including their fat classmates, in real life. Encouraging them to see the problematic nature of the language and the manipulation and editing of shows like the *Biggest Loser* by watching with a critical eye is one way to combat their negative impact on who we believe fat people are. Presenting kids with informational texts that counter normative narratives about health and wellness can open conversations about what we mean by healthy, and how we act it out. Aside from filters like the ones they can put on their social media photos, the ways that shows like this are produced are an illusion. Teaching students the warning signs of eating and exercise disorders in health and science classes should pair with conversations about how it shows up in our media whenever possible, even despite our best efforts as a culture to say we're not promoting a dangerous attainment of the thin ideal (we are).

According to the National Eating Disorders Association, symptoms of anorexia include: "Intense fear of gaining weight or becoming fat, even though underweight; being disturbed by one's shape or size enough to cause constant self-monitoring (weigh-ins, body checking), denial of the seriousness of low body weight, being preoccupied with weight, food, calories, fat grams, and dieting; refuses to eat certain foods, and often eliminates whole food groups (carbohydrates, fats, etc.); develops food rituals (eating foods in certain order, counting bites, or chews) and denies feeling hunger; expressing a need to 'burn off' calories eaten and engages in compensation behaviors around exercise; rigid and inflexible thinking style and has difficulty adapting to change."[206] Though anorexia is typically characterized by low weight and for this reason is the deadliest mental health condition, the strong presence of other symptoms paints a picture of anorexic behavior that is still dangerous even at a "normal" or high weight. All of these traits are present in the philosophy of *The Biggest Loser* and many of Michaels' other training programs. The only reason they have been culturally accepted is because of a cognitive dissonance built on the supposition that the alternative of "obesity" is far worse for one's health than a six-hour daily workout regimen (spoiler alert: it's not). In terms of physical symptoms, the body plummets into "starvation mode" after such periods of intense restriction, in which the body "expends fewer calories while waiting for food supplies to become plentiful again."[34, 205] While it is in this mode, it craves foods that Michaels demonizes regularly: fat and sugar, which help the body ride the wave of caloric deficit most efficiently.

Nutritionist Dr. Barry Sears[203] summarized the illusion of wellness provided by *The Biggest Loser*: "First, eating less can cause stress to the system causing more hunger. Second, the more people exercise, the hungrier they become." Dr. Sears continues by claiming that

> even with the most intense training, people are unlikely to add more than five pounds of muscle in 12 weeks of weight training. The reason viewers see their muscles emerging as the show goes on is because as the layer of fat surrounding the muscles is lost, muscles become more visible. Those muscles were always there but covered by a mass of fat tissue.[203]

The biggest indicator that *The Biggest Loser* is not at all about health, but about weight loss and the sensationalization of fat bodies for entertainment, is right in the disclosures they make in order to produce the show in the first place. Contestants must be over 18, have at least 80 pounds to lose, and are required to certify that they believe they are "in excellent physical, emotional, psychological and mental health."[201] Yet another contradiction exists here: the entire premise of the show is that being fat is an independent factor in lack of health and fitness. If contestants are in excellent health, why do they need Michaels for any other reason than to validate the cultural bias we have against fat bodies?

If these methods were healthy or safe, they also wouldn't need a warning label. And yet, at the end of each episode, a blurb appears on the screen:

Our contestants were supervised by doctors while participating in the show, and their diet and exercise regimen were tailored to their medical status and their specific needs. Consult with your own doctor before embarking on any diet or exercise program.

In 2016, the results of a long-term study by the U.S. National Institute of Health (NIH) were released that documented the weight gain and loss of contestants in Season 8 of the show, which aired in 2009. The study found that most of the 16 contestants regained their weight, and in some cases gained more than before they entered the contest – a fact that is often used in support of the argument that "diets don't work." The contestants' metabolism had overall slowed so dramatically that they were burning hundreds of calories a day less on average than people who weighed what they did at their "new" size after the show.[205] Since this study, many former contestants have advocated for the show to be canceled; it went on hiatus in 2016, but is back on U.S.A. Network as of 2020. Previous seasons are available to stream on Fandango at Home, Amazon Prime Video, and Apple TV.

Over the years, Michaels has advocated her own "Master Your Metabolism" diet, which involves a lot of commitment and a rigid set of food rules. On this diet, Michaels believes, disciples will lose weight, lower their cardiovascular risks, and lower risks for diabetes and cancer. The guidelines include:

◆ Eliminating hydrogenated fats, oils, refined grains, artificial sweeteners, and food dyes as well as starchy vegetables.

♦ Eat mostly foods she calls "power nutrients": beans and peas, onions and leeks, berries, meat and eggs, colorful produce, cruciferous and/or dark leafy green veggies, organic low-fat dairy (a half gallon of which costs $7 in 2024), and whole grains.

Of course, to maintain this plan, you can buy Michaels' cookbook, filled with recipes and tips. There's no cost other than the price of groceries, but Michaels offers an app with personalized weight loss advice starting at $14.99 per month.[207] In addition to this dietary plan, she recommends 4–5 hours of intense exercise weekly, which is two more hours than the standard recommendation for maintaining cardiovascular health.[208] In her own life, Michaels fasts for 12–14 hours a day and eats in the remaining hours.[126] She also puts heavy cream in her coffee, a ritual she calls "dirty fasting" because it involves consuming a food that she calls an "anti-nutrient."[202, 208] These methods, along with the rigidity required to abide by them, resemble anorexia and exercise bulimia. The terms "dirty fasting" and "anti-nutrient" are not widely accepted or used by nutrition or health science experts. Also worthy of note, that some of the foods Michaels hails as universally beneficial "power nutrients" (another pseudoscientific term) are harmful to those with hypothyroidism, namely cruciferous vegetables in high quantities, because they reduce the body's uptake of iodine, an element needed in the production of thyroid hormones. The danger of advice that is not based in science is that while it purports to be universally true, it can have adverse effects for many.

> **Quick Tip**
>
> *Invite students to research popular health claims and to find the proof that the claim is true or untrue using evidence and data.*

Another prominent figure in fitness culture is 22-year-old YouTuber Sam Sulek. In just three short years of lifting, he went from scrawny teen to 240-pound bodybuilder boasting 20-inch arms, which he measured in front of his massive audience.[209]

Sulek has garnered both praise and criticism, and has a following of 2.5 million users on TikTok and 3.5 million YouTube subscribers. His physique as well as his intense and extreme workout regimens and 7,000-calorie bulking diets (including donuts and chocolate milk) are the stuff of online intrigue and even memes. His content also serves as a model for young people – including those that I teach who follow him. He says proudly that the phrase "I'm too big" doesn't "exist in his vocabulary," and the speculation that he uses performance-enhancing drugs to maintain his build remains unanswered.[209, 210] With the normalization of symptoms of anorexia being both subtle and obvious in diet culture messaging, the presence of "bigorexia" is not hard to spot in most of Sulek's content. Still, even other bodybuilders worry about the influence he may be having on young people, who think that his extreme methods such as lifting high volume weights and doing lots of sets, even advocate lifting into "muscle failure," or the muscle's inability to contract concentrically.[211] Such workouts can lead to long and short-term injury and the need for more recovery time between workouts to avoid muscle overuse and atrophy.

For young people who are still developing their muscles, exercise of this intensity can be dangerous. Though people who defend Sam Sulek say that he can't be to blame if people copy him because "he's just showing us a day in his life," he offers direct advice to his audience during many of his videos about lifting. In one video, he gives a simple mantra: "Get a pump. Go to failure. Enjoy."[209] Just like the trend of science misinformation and monetization of content, students should know and investigate the ways that creators like Sulek (and thousands of others) are monetized on social media platforms in the same ways that athletes get endorsements to sell products for money; just like Denise Austin did for Reebok in the 1980s. To date, it's estimated that Sulek makes $2 million annually from posting his videos, including through YouTube and TikTok monetization as well as supplement sponsorships.[212] The throughline from getting people to doubt themselves and spend their money on products, diet scams, supplements is something that not even kids on social media are exempt from. Even I admit to falling for some of them. This is where our teachers play a significant role in seeing and stopping the problem: If students are able to interrogate the motivation behind the content they're seeing, they become more able to filter the facts from fiction and question the integrity of online content.

On average, U.S. teens spend most of their time on apps like YouTube, TikTok, and Instagram; and 37 percent of those teens use these apps, among others, for as many as five hours per day.[213] Among the highest frequency users of social media in this survey, 60 percent of them said their parents monitor their use very little, 25 percent said they had weak relationships with parents, and ten percent said they had poor mental health and reported feelings of suicidality. In my experience, adults don't monitor teen social media use not because they don't care what their kids are consuming, but because the generation gap combined with how fast social media is growing means they don't always know how to use it. It's difficult to keep up with a moving target. Not only should parents, teachers, and school leaders know what's happening online and in the media; but we must also be prepared to talk honestly and openly about it. Social media's power, for the good and the bad, is worth the attention of our school communities, especially when considering its impact on body image. When kids have the power to curate their feeds, they may do so in a way that "concentrate[s] exposure to content that perpetuates problematic norms about weight" while filtering out the content, images, and lived experiences of those at the margins.[214]

Better efforts at media literacy as well as building students' awareness around the frequency of media consumption could be a recipe for better resilience to filtered, edited, and fake news. They are used to hearing adults drone on about the horrors of screen time and social media; but leaning into the rise in its use is a chance to have conversations about what they're seeing, a chance to analyze it, and a chance to learn more about what they're seeing for ourselves. Developing their criticality as a skill is more than about critical thinking – it's critical thinking rooted in justice. "[Criticality] requires the ability to read, write, think, and speak in ways to understand power and equity in order to understand and promote anti-oppression as it relates to content areas."[176] Questions like *who's present/who's missing? Who's benefiting from this information?/Who isn't?* and *what is this asking me to think about/telling me to think or believe/convincing me to do/trying to make me feel?* can offer students new ways of thinking about the content they're seeing on their screens and in their world, and how it can help or harm their relationship to their bodies.

RUN IT BACK – Reflecting on Your Practice

Though models like the multi-period day or block scheduling make integrating content somewhat prohibitive – taking the time, space, and sharing the value of working together across curriculum is how we can most effectively notice when we are teaching diet culture, even when we don't mean to. Collaboration is key for spotting these inequities, as is knowing who in your department, administration, and among your colleagues is open to the work of seeing, stopping, and changing anti-fat bias. The more we are able to teach in and build community, the less inequity and body bias is likely to thrive because we can hold one another, and the units, lessons, and language we use accountable for "first, do no harm."

◆ *What does "first do no harm" mean to me, when talking about equity and teaching?*

◆ *How does weight stigma and diet culture remain a part of my content area?*

◆ *What cross-curricular relationships can I make to help students navigate diet culture and question narratives of anti-fat bias?*

◆ *What additional support do I need to unlearn anti-fat bias and lean toward equity in my own teaching? Who are the allies in my department, administration, and professional learning network?*

6

Cheeseburgers in Paradise

School Lunch, Food, and Diet Culture

The school cafeteria is easily one of the most overwhelming places in a school building. The pressure to "come in, eat, and leave" while also trying to decompress and socialize with friends is a jarring experience, and that's if you have a crew to sit with at all. Like academic content areas, many people and institutions (including the companies that provide it) see school lunch as a separate entity from children's learning; one that has nothing to do with education.[215]

Unpacking the Invisible Lunchbox

The transition from pyramid to plate is a result of a joint effort on behalf of the USDA and the U.S. Department of Health and Human Services. These two government organizations are required to provide reporting and necessary updates to American dietary guidelines every five years. The committee in charge of changing these guidelines has historically employed individuals with ties to companies like Novo Nordisk (Ozempic's Manufacturer), Dannon, the National Dairy Council, and Weight Watchers International.[216, 217]

DOI: 10.4324/9781003534143-8

Efforts to work with more local producers of food as opposed to frozen, ready-made products are on the rise, and this is promising. Before the pandemic, 42 percent of schools in America had "farm-to-school" programs.[215] According to an article by Jennifer Gaddis, author of *The Labor of Lunch: Why We Need Real Food and Real Jobs in Public Schools*, K-12 schools participating in farm-to-school programs

> redirected $789 million of public funding away from Big Food companies and into local food and farm economies, [seeking to] reclaim power from Big Food while also engaging K-12 students in agriculture-and garden-based experiences in which they learn about the food they eat and where it comes from.[215]

The pandemic brought on supply chain issues for major meal staples, making scratch-cooked school meals more of a challenge. Since 2020, budget constraints, inflation, and food availability have meant that some schools were not always abiding by USDA regulations in an effort to cut costs – but, of course, their corporate contractors stayed afloat. Tyson Foods made $43 billion in 2020, a $780 million *increase* in profit from the year before when there was no global health crisis.[218] Sodexo, a leading food service provider in schools, had a revenue of $1.9 billion, down 12 percent from the previous year.[219]

As a result, free school lunch programs opted less for hot meals and instead provided "grab and go" lunches, which included packaged snacks like Goldfish. What has come of the increase in packaged snacks and convenience foods is the rise of doubled-down diet culture and "my kid's not eating that" attitudes typically from middle-class parents. The cost of providing school meals depends on school size, average daily sales, and local labor and food markets. In an attempt to make nutritional access more widespread and equitable, the Healthy Hunger-Free Kids Act created regulations that address nutritional quality in schools and make nutritious meals more widely available to low-income families. According to the USDA, "Children may be determined 'categorically eligible' for free meals through participation in certain Federal Assistance Programs, such as the Supplemental Nutrition Assistance Program (SNAP), or based on their status as a homeless, migrant, runaway, or foster child."[220] In the 2024–2025 school year, a family of four earning $40,560 a year or less is eligible for free meals, and one earning $57,720 or less is eligible for reduced-price meals at school.[221]

"Free lunch" remains a stigmatizing label placed upon students from poor families – the same poor families often also seen as in need of weight intervention. "When lunch is free for everyone, the kids who need it aren't stigmatized by the kids who don't." But if lunch were free for everyone, how would corporations whose products are bartered within them turn a profit?

> As long as school meals continue to be a program that's just for lower income kids, it will still somehow always be okay for those meals not to be as high quality, which is horrible. But if we were to make it that all kids eat these meals, that actually might spur some governmental action to improve the overall quality of the meals.

said Priya Fielding-Singh, author of *How the Other Half Eats: The Untold Story of Food and Inequality in America*. Several states such as Colorado, Maine, Minnesota, New Mexico, California, New York, and Vermont have passed into law iterations of universal school lunch programs.[222] These differ from the extended and increased reimbursements provided through USDA federal initiatives that began with COVID. State governments have to opt in to the waiver before schools can serve free meals to all, but the waivers apply to breakfast and lunch at school.[223]

A school board in Waukesha, Wisconsin opted not to extend their COVID lunch-for-all programs after the pandemic, because they feared that this would make kids "addicted to free food" and "spoil" them.[223, 224] One school board member asserted that making free lunch more widely available would make families believe "it's someone else's problem to feed my children."[224] For as many as 12 million kids in the United States,[223] free breakfast and lunch are the only meals they have access to – and that, quite literally, is the school's problem. And it's our problem not just because they can focus better and behave better when they are fed; but because when schools care for students, focus and behavior are intrinsically easier to manage. Reporter Jessica Terrell says "One of the biggest barriers to improving the National School Lunch Program is that it is seen as charity rather than a public service." After the media uncovered public outcry in Wisconsin, the board reversed the decision.[225]

Conversations that blame foods, and poor people, rather than the corporations that take shortcuts are rooted in wellness, classism, and white supremacy cultures combined. The people who eat "cheap" food that is less nutrient dense are scapegoated, instead of placing blame on systems that make "healthy" food less affordable and available. People who can afford to eat plant-based or whole food diets (middle class, white Americans) can thus maintain their privileged status.

> Wellness culture is walking up and down a grocery store aisle, talking about unhealthy certain foods are because they're "cheap" and in packages, while simultaneously ignoring the accessibility of those nourishing foods and the prevalence of food insecurity and poverty,

said Shana Spence, an "all foods fit" dietitian known online as @thenutritiontea.[226] In her book *Eating While Black: Food Shaming and Race in America*, Psyche Williams-Forson states:

> Often, in today's public conversations, we focus almost solely on food access Who has access to "good" food? From where do they get it? Is the area affected by food apartheid? And so on. This aspect of food is certainly important, but it may come at the expense of ignoring other valuable aspects including habits, ideals and ideologies, quality, convenience, social and emotional frameworks, health and nutrition, location and disloca-tion, commensality and socializing.[227]

According to the UCONN Rudd Center for Food Policy and Health, local educational agencies and school districts that participate in the National School Lunch Program (free lunch) must establish a wellness policy,[228] committing to "promoting student wellness, preventing and reducing childhood obesity, and providing assurance that school meal nutrition guidelines meet the minimum federal school meal standards." Even then, the meals provided meet a bare minimum nutritional standard, while kids who can afford it get the highest levels of nutrition their money can buy. Kids on the "lowest rung" of federal feeding assistance programs still receive 16.8 pounds of food per week through the National School Lunch Program.[229]

And without weight stigma education and an understanding of the impression that fear of an "epidemic" leaves on our students, policies like this may pose the danger of emboldening schools to become places where "intervention" and diet culture play out on certain kids under the banner of "wellness." Requirements of these policies include that schools must outline "nutrition promotion and education, physical activity, and other school-based activities that promote student wellness." The NSLP school wellness plan rule also requires that they provide standards for all foods and beverages sold and not sold to students, including during classroom parties, classroom snacks brought in by parents, or food distributed "as incentives" by classroom teachers. The policies they draft mandate the management of food and beverage marketing, and a plan for public involvement and community partnerships.[230] Nothing is wrong with a wellness plan: but when it's crafted by adults and community members whose mission is to "do something about" the size of kids' bodies, it becomes less and less about wellness and more about moralizing food.

Additionally, in order to receive funding to feed kids, schools end up policing the food that kids eat during school hours. Such responsibility falls on whoever the "wellness policy leadership" is – and that person, according to the USDA, should "have the authority and responsibility to ensure each school complies with the policy."[230] It becomes another way of disciplining the most vulnerable kids in the classroom and the cafeteria through a culture of shame, perceived ignorance, assumptions, and fatphobia. Williams-Forson says that "The practices of shaming and policing

Black people's bodies with and around food arise from a broader history of trying to control our very states of being, and this assumed stance is rooted in privilege and power."[227] She argues that the monitoring of marginalized people, especially Black people, and the food they eat, "aids in the idea that Black people are in more general need of regulation, correction and control."

The regulations outlined in the Healthy, Hunger-Free Kids Act of 2010 illustrate conflicting narratives about what we imagine "health" is in general, from a public policy perspective. Food giants had the incentive to make their foods less caloric by the 2014 school year, thus villainizing the calorie and spotlighting calorie reduction as giving the *appearance* of health.[215, 231] And as I mentioned in Chapter 4, the FDA still allows for a significant margin of error on nutrition fact labels, which renders this caloric change not only marginal, but potentially not even completely accurate. Whether their food is "healthy" or not, the role of massive corporations in schools remains ethically, not necessarily dietarily, problematic because their aim is largely not kids' health, but their profit margin. And rather than successfully aim to reduce the tremendous role of these food corporations in our school cafeteria altogether, the White House empowered them to change their product (negligibly) in order to have continued influence over the student-consumer market. Undoubtedly all food fits and has value – but I'm left wondering: were any of the vendors contracted to feed our students required to commit to meaningfully doing anything to reduce environmental and public health problems within these communities? Are they teaching them to have a relationship with their bodies other than "buy our stuff, but don't get fat?"

If the answer is no, then what we have is programming predicated on performing rather than *being* healthy: which is again conflated with eating less and achieving thinness as a proxy for health.

A 2018 analysis of 16 years of data concluded that schools "are now the single healthiest place Americans are eating,"[232] probably owing to the Obama Administration's efforts to change nutritional quality in schools. In general, the USDA purchases between 15 and 20 percent of all the foods that make up lunches served at school; schools mostly use the program to get lean meat and produce. Of the foods that make up school lunches, 15 to 20 percent are purchased by the U.S. Department of Agriculture through its "Foods in Schools" program. School districts mostly use the program to get lean meat and produce.[232] Even Michelle Obama's campaign and the federal laws that bolstered it were not free from the burden of corporate interest and weight stigma. In an effort to extend Let's Move! Into the school cafeteria, Michelle Obama helped change the availability of packaged snacks in school cafeterias across the United States. As a stipulation of the bill, the "Smart Snacks in Schools," rule placed limits on the amount of fat, sugar, sodium, and calories of à la carte foods sold during the school day.[215] Aubrey Gordon also explains it in her book:

> Let's Move! was bolstered by corporate food producers with a stake in maintaining a status quo that bolstered sales of their products. Companies like Coca-Cola, Hershey's, Kraft, and Kellogg's signed onto the First Lady's healthy weight commitment...agreeing to reformulate their foods to become "healthier" – that is, less caloric. Ultimately, many of those changed foods only resulted in minor calorie reductions (ten or twenty calories per portion) and offered corporations a new marketing platform that appeared to give their products the White House's seal of approval.[17]

Quick Tip

Ask students to pay closer attention to their school lunch options. Ask and answer the following criticality questions together:

◆ *What brands are available to us in the cafeteria? How do those brands make our food and treat our environment?*

◆ *How do the goals of certain brands (getting us to buy) compare and contrast to our school's messages about what "healthy" means?*

◆ *What stereotypes exist about school lunch that we need to examine more closely? Where do these ideas come from?*

Must Be the Money (Again)

The food and beverage industry (McDonald's, Coca-Cola, etc.) spent $27 million in 2020 lobbying Congress, and $15 million as of the summer of 2024. The top spender on lobbying during this election cycle is Coca-Cola at over $2.5 million.[233] One leading lobby is Aramark, a food service company used widely in schools and prisons across America – which in 2023 spent $330,000 lobbying and in 2024 so far has spent $180,000 on lobbying.[234] In 2012, roughly 80 percent of schools in America had a contract with Coca-Cola or Pepsi.[235] Schools have signed these contracts in the last twenty years in an effort to save money, opting less often for scratch-cooked meals and more frequently relying on freezer-to-oven prep. In an episode of the *LEFT OVER* Podcast, reporter and host Jessica Terrell states that:

> Aramark is one of three companies – along with Compass Group and Sodexo – collectively known as "the Big Three" in the food service industry. In 2019, the last full year before the pandemic, "the Big Three" earned a combined $40 billion in the United States. The activists who created the first school-meals programs in the 1900s fought hard to keep for-profit businesses out of school cafeterias. It's a fight they lost at the inception, and expansion, of the National School Lunch Program. Today, private companies exercise vast control over what students eat, how it gets on their plates, and even who serves it to them.[236]

She also noted that in the United States there are only six states where no school district contracts with private companies: Louisiana, Alabama, Hawaii, Kentucky, West Virginia, and North Dakota.[236] When she reached out to representatives in California, Texas, and New York, they either didn't respond or said they don't track the number of districts using corporate food companies to feed their kids – which I find curious, because these states track something as personal as BMI data, but don't know how schools are feeding students?

The influences of corporations and government food initiatives have made it so that advertisements for products are a regular part of our kid's school day, too. Those posters with famous people donning milk mustaches and equally famous two-word phrases are a product of government "checkoff programs," also known as "research and promotion" campaigns.[237, 238] These ads exist for the same reason you see Hass avocados marketed as the new and trendy "superfood," and stuffed crust pizzas from Domino's every other commercial while streaming your favorite shows – government checkoff programs funded such marketing campaigns in an effort to sell more than 12 million pounds of cheese in 2023.

Negativity about the word "processed" is often led by a misguided fear rooted in diet culture. The word "processed" has garnered negative connotation and been used to talk about food so much that we have strayed away from what we mean when we use this language to discuss the way food is made. Cooking is a way of "processing" foods, too. Words like "processed" and "GMO" have become ways to place certain foods on a moral high ground (or not), and the anxiety around "processed foods" at school is less about what's in it and more about how it's made. Due to the increase in cost-saving corporate relationships as opposed to scratch-cooked meals, food at school is often made in factories, frozen, and then shipped or trucked across state lines, and reheated in the school's kitchen. The amount of travel our food has to do to get to our kids' lunch trays makes it less nutrient dense *and* less appetizing.[239] Certain temperatures (frozen to hot, for example) alter the molecular nutritional value of the food – and that is where "processing" is cause for concern. The 2024 Final Rule Requirements for school meal programs passed a "Buy American" proposal amendment to school meal regulations, which would reduce non-domestically grown products to five percent of a school's food product procurement. Schools agreed to a "phase in" approach rather than an immediate adherence to the five percent rule, meaning that by 2026, schools must cut down non-domestically grown and produced foods they serve to ten percent, then eight percent by 2029, then five percent by

2032.[240] The changes also *allow*, but do not *require*, schools to procure "locally grown," "locally raised," or "locally caught" foods, effective in the summer of 2024.

The lack of responsibility that corporations have to the environment around them is appalling, and should be enough to make schools question who they're doing business with. One disturbing case of the contradictions between health, food, and disease is happening in two counties in North Carolina.[241] In Duplin and Sampson counties, there are about as many hogs for slaughter as there are people – and their presence has created an environmental justice issue of large proportions. Smithfield, a large producer of pork products, constructed the largest hog slaughterhouse in the world in nearby Bladen county.[242, 243, 237] Most of these farms are situated in low-income communities of color, and their "waste pit lagoons" create biogas, "dirty" energy generated from the pigs' urine and feces.[242] Even with laws restricting swine farms from being built close to residences, schools, hospitals, and churches,[244, 245] the waste from pigs leeches into local water supply, and farmers water their grass with it. This produces not only air and water pollution but also a stench that stretches for miles. Such practices have created high levels of asthma, sinus problems and cancer in residents living nearby. Even after a 1997 moratorium on "lagoon-farms" was signed into law, Hurricane Floyd displaced water from existing farms and contaminated the water supply just two years later.[243] Residents have brought complaints before the EPA on the basis of civil rights.[243]

The case of Duplin and Sampson counties illuminates that Black Americans are subject to racial discrimination via food apartheid, housing inequity, and environmental racism; but, as Dr. Williams-Forson asserts, they are not "helpless pawns": they are aware, in cases like this, that they are being poisoned, and know what it takes to make these products, and many refrain from eating them because of it.[246, 237] The positioning of Black bodies as "needing intervention" and "lacking education" about food, when they quite literally live in the belly of the factory farming beast, is a racist assumption – one that Ibram Kendi says is predicated on "beliefs about Black inferiority" which lead to "racial ideas that are designed to legitimize racial inequality, racist policies, and divisions, because those who perpetuate this kind of misinformation most often benefit from its psychic and social power."[227] And it's one that our school lunch rooms and federal initiatives to "intervene" in childhood "obesity" force them to internalize. Black people have always exhibited culinary creativity and genius, despite the systems that compromise their social and physical determinants of health. Williams-Forson quotes literary scholar Barbara Christian, who states that

> I have students, both black and white, who believe these [negative] images because it is become a thread throughout major fiction, film, popular culture...It is become a part of our psyche. It's a real indication that one of the best ways of maintaining a system of oppression has to do with psychological control of people.[227]

In his first 100 days of his second term, President Trump also gutted EPA regulations that would address environmental racism like the kind happening in North Carolina hog farming country, by walking back the 1994 Clinton executive order 12,898, a directive that sought to make addressing environmental racism a priority in all government agencies, beginning with "the 1982 designation of a small, mostly Black community in Warren County, North Carolina as the site of a hazardous waste landfill intended for soil contaminated by toxic waste illegally dumped along state roadways."[247] According to President Trump, this executive order is "DEI," and to address policies in place to protect communities of color from environmental harm is "discriminatory," "illegal," and "preferential."[248] Ironically, the same administration is not concerned that wealthy, predominantly white communities who have clean air and water are being treated "preferentially," and are okay with those things being a privilege only afforded to some. It's only "discriminatory" when people of color fight back or are granted some justice.

> **Quick Tip**
>
> In etymological (word study), scientific, mathematical, and historical contexts, ana-
> lyze what the word "processed" means when we talk about food. Some teaching
> ideas:
>
> ◆ How far does the food in the cafeteria travel to get to our school?
> ◆ What kinds of cooking methods are used to prepare different foods?
>   (poaching, broiling, baking, etc.)
> ◆ How does temperature (storage, cooking, etc.) affect the nutrient density of
>   different foods?
> ◆ What biases do we need to investigate about people who eat "processed"
>   foods?
> ◆ What connotation does the word processed have as it relates to food, and
>   why?

In a 2011 response to the increase in cost-effective foods in schools, Congress met to discuss a spending bill that would alter USDA regulations on vegetable servings in school-provided meals, keeping french fries and pizza on the menu. Potato growers and food companies that produced frozen pizzas requested the changes, and Republican advocates for the bill agreed that telling students what to eat at school was government overreach and would "prevent overly burdensome and costly regulations and to provide greater flexibility for local school districts to improve the nutritional quality of meals."[249]

Eventually, Congress declared that half a cup of tomato paste on pizza served in schools counted as a serving of vegetables. The intentions behind initiatives to shift school lunches became clearer with this debate on Capitol Hill…and also highlights the crossover of military recruitment in poor, rural communities and communities with large populations of BIPOC students with the desire to make kids "healthier" – thus, more fit for military service. According to a 2011 article for NBC,

A group of retired generals advocating for healthier school lunches also criticized the spending bill. The group, called Mission: Readiness has called poor nutrition in school lunches a national security issue because obesity is the leading medical disqualifier for military service.[(249)]

The language of the "security threat" posed by "obesity," thus inevitably made its way to the school cafeteria – and conflated nutrition and health with thinness, again.

In my research on the "pizza is a vegetable" controversy that I remember hearing as a high school student, I couldn't help but wonder if politicians were actually responding to the wrong problem. Vilifying fries and pizza, both valid sources of nutrition, is a function of diet culture rooted in a fear of becoming fat; and yet, the link between this anti-deliciousness witch hunt and the government's desire to recruit more soldiers is unsurprising.

Despite the fact that school lunches are, as it turns out, relatively healthy, what if kids are opting for fries and pizza because the "healthy" options aren't palatable? Some kids spend upwards of $40 a week on packaged a la carte snacks.[(225)] A research survey of 23 faculty and staff and 26 students at a New England school in 2000 – despite the fact that schools must adhere to USDA guidelines for the National School Breakfast and Lunch Programs, food is less appealing and palatable to students in cafeterias – so they opt for the snack stand or packaged foods instead.[(5)] In my own experience, I generally avoided school lunch except for a daily bagel with butter in elementary school, because nothing else tasted or even looked appealing on the lunch line. I stopped buying lunch in high school after years of rubbery chicken patties, lukewarm chocolate milk, and canned, soggy vegetables soaked in brine – all foods that are considered "healthy," but are prepared in a mass-production format that aims to feed lots of kids, fast – and in doing so, may compromise their appeal to the very kids they're feeding. What if, instead of telling kids what to eat from a place of food shame, we transformed what they eat so they'd *actually want to eat it*?

And how often are the foods that are representative of the cultures of kids who attend the school actually on the menu? A consequence of the USDA MyPlate guidelines is that they are also not inherently culturally responsive, which may lead some kids to feel shame about their favorite cultural foods. As we saw in earlier chapters, deciding what foods are "good" and "bad" is not politically, morally, or even racially neutral. Psyche Williams-Forson aptly states:

> Everyone, from pundits to journalists, food scholars... seems to have some expertise on what is considered "fresh," "healthy" and "wholesome" food for all people...Eating is no longer just about enjoying your food but assigning labels: "organic," "sustainable," "healthy," "clean" and "local." And at the heart of this culinary madness is often an attitude of moral certitude that one person, or group of persons, is more knowledgeable on what everyone else should be eating, as well as when, where, and why.[227]

Putting up posters in the cafeteria with MyPlate guidance may encourage universalization that excludes kids and their dietary restrictions, cultural customs, and identities. In these guidelines, we miss opportunities for cultural curiosity and connection; what do kids who eat halal or kosher eat like? What are some delicious combinations of foods they can try?

And if those menus become more culturally responsive and feature dishes that reflect the cultures and identities of the kids who eat them, it can give kids who do not share those identities exposure to new foods, too. Even better – inviting parents who make these dishes at home from the heart and from memory, rather than following an unfamiliar recipe, is an invitation to the community that signals that feeding kids is everyone's business, and that their lives, their joy, their nourishment, and their academic success are not separate. "Food is NOT just about calories. It can be culture, nourishment, self-care, love, fun, hope, and friendship – all in one," tweeted Dr. Chukwuemeka Nwuba, a London-based eating disorder specialist.[250]

Josh Goddard, head of nutrition at a school district in Santa Ana, California, argues that while manufacturers can make cultural foods for schools easily, reflecting the "rich and meaningful culinary traditions of Latino families that make up a majority of the students in the district" can't really happen "without cooking food locally." In a podcast interview with Jess Terrell,

To assume we can delegate that to a manufacturer, right. And that a pizza or a perfect tamale is going to show up that exactly reflects our local identity, we're dreaming. We have to do it ourselves. So it is this idea of self-determination, right? That we have to be guided by.[225]

Along these lines, the 2024 school meal Final Rule update also included a passed proposal that includes that traditional indigenous foods can be served as part of a reimbursable school meal, which is a start[240] – but available and reimbursable does not necessarily mean enthusiastically celebrated or destigmatized. "Food is cultural and deeply personal," says Oona Miller Hanson,

And add in any number of special considerations (food allergies, eating disorders, GI conditions, physiological differences, etc.) and what makes sense for one kid doesn't apply at all to another. One-size-fits-all lessons about nutrition just don't make sense, and they can end up doing a lot of harm.[62]

Kids can leave the cafeteria getting informal lessons on how they eat is "wrong," or "bad."

In fact, while it is making room for more "local" and indigenous food practices, food policy as it relates to school meals is still very much shaped around the regulation and "intervention" upon racialized bodies. In addition to the assumptions made about Black health and wellness, and the need for surveillance of the "obese" Black child in the physical education setting, this fixation and assumption of Black ignorance about food and health pervades the lunchroom, too. "We do not need social media or anything/anyone else to tell us what, how and when to eat," says Psyche Williams-Forson.[227] The effort to "intervene" in the eating habits of youth of color specifically is often grounded in white saviorism and racial and cultural stereotypes about what Black people eat and what we think they know about health.

When these sentiments are couched in offers of community improvement – such as building gardens, helping children reduce obesity, or embracing a particular way of eating to conjure a healthier lifestyle – they are difficult to identify as belonging to an anti-Black or a white supremacist agenda.

Williams-Forson unpacks the "nice white racism" of food and health policy initiatives, and suggests that even ones purported by Black people (like Mrs. Obama) are not necessarily benevolent, either.

"The physical action of Black people consuming food," she says, is seen as, in itself, a transgression. She continues,

> From incendiary and denigrating images of African Americans with chicken and watermelon, to policies that suggest African Americans have the worst health records, to arguments that food is the culprit in our early deaths, racist ideas are continuously contrived in order to try and convince us and society at large of Black inferiority. This is just one of the many ways that white supremacy works to maintain power structures' it creates hysteria where no actual threat exists in order to justify surveilling, controlling and killing Black people with impunity.[227]

Bulls on Parade

Maintaining diet culture is very much political. Moralizing food and even entire food groups has led to a hysteria around food dyes and additives, which Secretary Robert F. Kennedy Jr. has claimed are "linked to cancer and ADHD." During the Biden administration, red dye no. 3 was banned after cancer studies were done in rats. Under Kennedy's direction, The FDA recently announced that food producers will need to stop using synthetic food dyes by the end of next year. These ingredients include Red No. 40, Yellow No. 5, Yellow No. 6, and Green No. 3.[231, 232] The natural alternatives slated for approval, which include red algae, have not been proven to be safe alternatives – yet. The evidence that red dye is connected to ADHD is tenuous at best, despite the secretary's claim that the studies indicate a "very very strong link." In a speech in West Virginia, he said:

> So the loneliness, the dispossession, the crisis that we have in mental health, in suicide, in ADD, ADHD, all of these are linked – and particularly to the dyes...It's very clear the dyes that Gov. Morrisey is banning, all of them are linked in very, very strong studies to ADHD and to cancers. So we're seeing an explosion in cancers in this country.[(253)]

As a matter of fact, "The only food additives for which evidence has shown a link with cancer are nitrites and nitrates, which are used as preservatives in processed meat," the American Institute for Cancer Research states on its website. "Eating processed meat is strongly associated with an increased risk of colorectal cancer. There is currently no other strong evidence linking food additives to an increased cancer risk."[(254)] The concern about food dyes in their current form comes from the fact that they are "petroleum based," which, we've established, does not mean the same as eating gasoline. The presence of some compounds in one form does not make them dangerous in others by default.

Nevertheless, RFK and his narrative persist – people are lonely and "dispossessed" not because of rising food and housing costs, or lack of connection and defunding mental health services – but because of red food dye. In the same visit to West Virginia, RFK also publicly fat-shamed the governor while standing behind a placard that read "MAHA Starts Here," and offered to do a public weigh in once he'd lost thirty pounds on his next visit.[(255)] West Virginia has the second lowest life expectancy rate in America, and is notorious for a widespread opioid epidemic and some of the highest overall poverty and childhood poverty rates in the country. Still, West Virginia's Governor Patrick Morrissey plans to implement the "Four Pillars of a Healthy West Virginia," which includes banning food dyes in public school lunches, "expanding the current mandatory employment and training requirements" for SNAP eligibility, emphasizing movement, and "rewarding healthy food choices."[(256)] Once again, politicians put the onus on the poorest people with the most needs to "make America healthy again." Over 183,000 (67 percent) of the students in West Virginia are eligible for free or reduced lunch. I don't know about you, but I don't think it's the food dyes that are "dispossessing" them and their parents.[(257)]

The same leader who is demonizing foods is also standing by while colleagues in the Congress and Senate make access to food more difficult for the poorest of Americans. In the budget proposal colloquially known as the "Big Beautiful Bill," Republican representatives posed a $300 billion cut to SNAP and WIC to give tax breaks to the wealthy. U.S. Senate Committee on Agriculture, Nutrition, and Forestry projects that "420,000 children each month will see decreased National School Lunch Program and School Breakfast Program assistance due to the state cost shifts, as interconnections between SNAP and school meals."[(258)] Congress passed the bill in July of 2025, and still stands to cut off 17 million people from their healthcare as of this writing in addition to the cuts to nutrition for children.

Though the mission to "Make America Healthy Again" hasn't taken on as much blatant anti-fat rhetoric as previous administrations, it does not mean it's absent. After all, the legacy that Kennedy, Jr. follows is one of words like "vigor" and "fitness" being used to push anti-fat policy and practice everywhere from school to parenting and beyond. So far, (and this chapter is being written just six months into Trump's presidency), it sounds like "chronic disease," a supposed "autism epidemic" and "health." But history tells us that "making America healthy again" means that some people will make the cut, and others will have their benefits – the very ones that help them achieve health – cut. Upon his confirmation, he promised America that he would not take away our Diet Coke or Twinkies, "which [his boss] loves." Right there is an admission that the eugenicist rhetoric to come was meant for us, the regular people, and not for anyone in power.[(259)] In West Virginia and nationwide, the wealthy and powerful will get to keep their sugary drinks and foods – while the rest of us are personally blamed for being fat, poor, and "dispossessed."

Since the second term of President Donald Trump and the hiring of Robert F. Kennedy, Jr. as the Secretary of Health and

Human Services, the outlook expressed by people like Bonnie Prudden, and even by his believed-to-be-more-progressive late uncle, remain similarly oppressive and problematic. At his own confirmation hearing, Robert F. Kennedy Jr. referred to obesity (and, by extension, fat people) as an "existential threat to America."[260] He has even gone as far to suggest that "parental obesity" could be a cause of autism, and voted to study it, along with "mold and food additives" as a potential cause.[261] The problem here, from a scientific and data interpretation perspective, is that it takes a small kernel of a supposed truth, that parental "obesity," especially that of maternal fatness, is to blame for kids who develop autism. According to the American Academy of Pediatrics (AAP):

> A case-control study of autism spectrum disorders (ASDs) in California recently demonstrated that mothers who were obese before pregnancy had a 67% increase in risk of having children with ASDs. Other studies have found that children of obese mothers have an increased occurrence of attention-deficit/hyperactivity disorder symptoms, an increased risk of intellectual disability (IQ <70), lower mean scores on cognitive testing, and a higher risk of schizophrenia later in life.[262]

Based on this single medical conclusion, the leader of Health and Human Services has purported the idea that fat moms cause autism. But, as we know, correlation and causation are not the same, and risk factors are not causes. Further in the paper's results, it states: "The association between maternal prepregnancy obesity and child cognition is not consistent across studies; some studies have found no such associations."[262]

In a SiriusXM Radio interview, Secretary Kennedy said that "If the autism epidemic was an artifact … of new changing diagnostic criteria or better recognition, you would see it in all age groups." According to Fact Check, the increase can be attributed to screening, for which "medical and governmental recommendations and policies encouraged diagnosis in younger generations without providing similar pathways or incentives for those who were already adults to get diagnosed."[263] Kennedy also claimed early on in the second Trump term that they would "find the cause of autism by September [2025]," which is a gross misunderstanding of how the scientific method works. Deadlines don't exist for scientific discovery, and the point of creating a hypothesis is to repeatedly prove it, gather new information, and draw conclusions based on what you see – not on what you hope the outcome will be. Science doesn't draw the conclusions you want out of thin air, especially not on demand. Still, he said in a half-hour press conference that research regarding the genetic factors that play a role in fetal development, especially those related to autism prognosis, is a "dead end."[264] From here, it's obvious that pushing a narrative, not scientific inquiry, is the priority.

And science certainly cannot advance when politicians cut the federal health research workforce by 25 percent, or by cutting billions from nutrition programming.[265] He claims, despite evidence that autism is largely genetic, that it is a "preventable disease" that "destroys families," comes from an "environmental toxin" that has been "released" into our food, air, and environment.[266] The thing about autism is that it's not a disease, it's a developmental condition. Kennedy, however, insists that it's an "epidemic."[264] Kennedy expounded on the claim even further, suggesting that "kids were fully functional" and then regressed to "full blown autism" because of some "environmental exposure into autism when they were two years old."[263, 264] According to the *New York Times*, "Scientists have not ruled out the possibility that both genes and environmental factors could influence whether a child develops autism. Still, there is no evidence to suggest that autism can be avoided."[264] Yet, what we know about autism suggests that kids don't just regress overnight; and that, for many, masking and social performance mean they go untested, unscreened, and untreated for many years, even into adulthood. Autism affects people of all ages, sizes, races, classes, and abilities.

Enveloped in this bias also is his feeling that autistic people, especially children, are somehow equally threatening to our society because of their perceived lack of ability to contribute to our economy. Also important to note that there is overlap in disability and fatness, just as there is with race and size, gender and size, and so on. Many autistic children are fat because the only foods they find palatable or not a sensory nightmare are those considered "processed." This kind of rhetoric used to demonize and otherize fat people, or anyone with a chronic condition, is stigmatizing at best and deadly at worst. Deadly because, when coupled with the defunding of public healthcare projects like Medicare and Medicaid and the positioning of health as a ways and means to achieve global superpower, the policies leave those who can't achieve health behind. MAHA culture and bootstrap culture are one and the same; it is one's personal responsibility, and thus their own personal failure, if they are too sick, too poor, too fat, or too marginalized. It lets the system be entirely free from criticism, and as a result, those same systems can go on harming marginalized people, including kids at school.

Since his failed presidential campaign, Kennedy has advocated for lower healthcare costs, and in doing so, goes after Big Pharma and food industry giants. On his campaign website, he made the claim that "When John F. Kennedy was president, 6% of American kids had a chronic health condition. Today it is 60%." He also promised to implement a national fitness program like the one his uncle started.[(267)] Even from his position today, he envisions a future where "autism is very rare," and has gone on record to state that people with obesity, autism, and chronic conditions did not exist or were not visible when he was growing up. "One hundred and 20 years ago, when somebody was obese, they were sent to the circus," Kennedy said. "There were literally case reports done about them. Obesity was almost unknown."[(268)] Kennedy claims that he rarely met anyone with a chronic condition growing up, despite being surrounded by family members who struggled with them. This kind of language is unmistakably related to eugenics, because it points to a history like the one discussed in Chapter 4, where fat and disabled people did in fact exist – they just disappeared because they were "ugly" and they were deemed "lesser" than thin people. The Venn diagram of reasons that those in power seek to erase disabled people and the reasons they seek to erase fat people is actually just a circle; people view both as disposable, especially in "Western" societies.

Robert F. Kennedy also conveniently ignores that his own late uncle and former President suffered from Addison's disease, a chronic condition, and took as many as 12 medications at once to manage several health problems throughout his life.[269] His aunt Eunice also had Addison's disease, and his aunt Rosemary underwent a controversial lobotomization at just 23 years old for depression. As early as his presidential campaign, he blamed "chronic illness" for rising healthcare costs, including those attributed to mental health and blamed it on the "Big Pharma Wall Street firms that control much of the medical industry" in order to "get richer."[267] And he wasn't wrong…but what often comes of this kind of language, especially from people with more than a billion dollars in generational wealth, is that the blame falls on those who don't have the ability to pay for healthcare costs out of pocket.

Diet culture as a politically unifying force becomes even more apparent when we examine the ways that both Michelle Obama and Robert F. Kennedy Jr. view "childhood obesity." Kennedy, like Mrs. Obama, wants to see children lose weight the old fashioned way, through "lifestyle changes" and diet and exercise. At the launch of her Plezi Nutrition organization and brand, she stated that:

> I winced when I saw the latest guidance for the medical community that came out a couple months ago – that in addition to eating healthier and being active, doctors are now advised to consider medication and surgery for kids over 12 when lifestyle changes aren't enough.[270]

Her problem isn't that the AAP guidelines are focused on telling fat kids they need to "fix" or "solve" the "problem" of their fatness, but that they're allowing kids to get surgery to do so. Why not choose instead to accept body diversity as a natural fact, and end the conversation that equates weight and size to health?

Robert F. Kennedy expresses similar sentiments when asked about GLP-1 and other weight loss drugs, which he has been vehemently against – a move that stands in opposition to his counterpart, Dr. Mehmet Oz. Kennedy said in a Fox News interview in October that pharma companies are counting on selling the drugs to Americans because "we're so stupid and so addicted to drugs." His plan, instead, is to implement fitness programming at a national level and change what's in our food. He said, "If we just gave good food, three meals a day, to every man, woman and child in our country, we could solve the obesity and diabetes epidemic overnight."[271] While these are noble and important intentions, they cannot happen without addressing disproportionate access to safe play spaces for kids, food deserts, and lack of equity across housing, food access, education, and other social necessities. All of these are things that the government exists to provide, and all are things that the president he works for is looking to gut through budget cuts, executive orders, and bad policy. Making America Healthy Again begins with investing in our social good, because there's more to health than personal responsibility.

Wanting kids to be healthier is not a bad thing. But unwaveringly equating size with health, and emphasizing personal responsibility as the way to do that without challenging or changing the environmental and economic factors that make peoples' lack of health possible is worth questioning. Michelle Obama is often credited with reducing childhood obesity by 43 percent, but the cost, in many cases, is their self-worth and an indictment of their families, specifically mothers with fewer resources.

At the start of the program, Mrs. Obama admitted that "I thought to myself, if a Princeton-and Harvard-educated professional woman doesn't know how to adequately feed her kids, then what are other parents going through who don't have access to the information I have?"[270, 272, 273]

It is important not to discount that Mrs. Obama has faced abject scrutiny for many of her successes, especially and often solely for being an educated, successful, and driven Black woman with proximity to power. In an article blasting the program, Daren Bakst from the right-wing think tank Heritage Foundation referred to Michelle's efforts as "arrogance on display."[273] The article continues to state that "attending Ivy-League schools doesn't magically make someone better parent material than an individual who attended a public university, or, dare it be said, someone who didn't attend college."[357] She didn't state anywhere in this quote that it made her more fit to make decisions about what kids eat at school – it was an admission that feeding kids a balanced diet is challenging for everyone, including those with proximity to wealth. If nothing else, it reveals that the pervasiveness of diet culture does not exclude even the most social-justice focused, well-intentioned people like the former First Lady. The articles published by Bakst dig even further at Mrs. Obama, and repeatedly used the "angry Black woman" trope, saying any critics inside the federal government have felt the "wrath" and "ire" of Mrs. Obama for having criticisms of her policies. There are valid criticisms to be made about the ways that diet culture showed up in these programs, and it is possible and necessary to make said criticisms without attacking Mrs. Obama or her husband.[270]

Mrs. Obama refers repeatedly in her introduction of the Partnership for a Healthier America to childhood obesity as a "threat," but does not mention the factors that she says contribute to the potential for "one third of all children born in 2000 or later" suffering from "diabetes…or chronic obesity-related health problems like heart disease, high blood pressure, cancer and asthma."[274] Also embedded into statements like this one are the conflation of correlation with causation, a common misstep that fuels anti-fat bias and healthism. There is also no mention of the fact that childhood asthma and cancer are often related to the built environment where children grow up, especially related to air quality. The PFHA overview also states that: "Rather than award grants, engage in policy discussions, or develop programmatic activities, the Partnership concentrates on mobilizing leadership from across sectors and at every level to take action that can have a significant impact on organizational goals."[274] Here, again, the language of individualism shows up even in the solutions; rather than putting economic power behind health or environmental justice, it's up to individual leaders to shift "organizational goals." The language of diet culture is also the language of corporatism. It calls on chefs, school officials, healthcare providers, and parents to do things like increase opportunities for physical activity in their communities, but retains little mention of how elected officials, those in power, can help shift the built environment. There are some suggestions including "form a community coalition tasked with identifying local barriers to healthy living," and "work with local childcare providers and after-school programs to implement evidence-based standards for nutrition, physical activity and screen time within childcare settings," For many communities, the issue is not a lack of desire to see healthier kids – it's a lack of economic power and the privilege of time to challenge those "local barriers."

Equating health to a matter of personal responsibility is the "bootstraps theory" of school lunch, and it's true that the Obama Administration did emphasize personal responsibility and parenting in a lot of its messaging. Though these initiatives got a lot wrong by leaning into the conservative values of individualism more often than not, it's not "government overreach" to turn the intention to care for one another into policy, and to make sure that wider varieties of foods are available to students. Ad hominem criticisms like those of the Heritage Foundation are unmistakably tied to the racism of watching Black people be in positions of power, and do something with that power to attempt to address issues; even if those efforts are misguided by diet culture and learned anti-fatness. None of us are immune to the oppressive paternalism that is anti-fat bias.

Come Together – A Case for "All Foods Fit"

The politics of food in general makes plain the ways that nutritional policy and food/body shame play out in all areas of a school and in their larger communities. Due to these corporate entanglements, combined with the explicit and implicit moralizing of entire food groups, schools are sending kids mixed messages constantly about food, their bodies, and what they should do with them – and there are entire industries providing and profiting off of that confusion. Researchers from the UCONN

Rudd Center for Food Policy and Health assert that "When we send our children to school, we expect them to learn about math, reading, and science. But food companies are also trying to teach them about their brands."[275] The very agencies creating guidelines that are supposed to make school meals more nutrient dense frequently prioritize corporate bottom lines over nutrition. Their efforts are not only to keep promoting their products and receiving funding and government subsidies to make sales, but to rail against climate change, too – an equity problem linked to their mass production efforts.[276] School meals and the distance they have to travel are also not environmentally sustainable, even when it is economical.

Advancing toward equity means that nutrition at school *must* be free of food *and* body shame. Ending food shame *and* increasing access to nutrition, however, won't happen by demonizing foods like fat, carbs, and sugar. Calling "obesity" a death sentence while making a boogeyman out of their favorite mac and cheese isn't how we get kids to be healthy – it's how we get them to be afraid. It's also how we maintain the oppressive tradition of placing food, and subsequently, people, on a hierarchy.

"That food being labeled as 'bad,' 'junk,' or 'unhealthy' might be one of the few safe foods for a child with an eating disorder or other medical condition," said Oona Hanson in a 2022 X post.[277] Shaming kids for bringing, buying. and eating the few safe foods they have just because it's bagged and "processed" doesn't help them heal their relationship to food. Nearly 3.2 percent of American children struggle with avoidant-restrictive food intake disorder or ARFID, which is often dismissed as "picky eating," but can have consequences for long-term health especially for kids in growing bodies. This disorder often onsets by age 12, but can begin as early as age six. According to Equip Health, "ARFID has serious consequences including heart problems, weak bones, hormonal disruptions, stunted growth, development of other mental health problems, and more."[278] A large number of kids with ARFID includes a disproportionate number of autistic and neurodivergent kids because they are sensitive to sensory input such as texture, flavor, and temperature. For kids with restrictive eating disorders, any calories are a good start and any nutrition is paramount while they are learning to explore foods that feel safe to eat. "Fed is best" is a general rule that *all* kids can benefit from (with the exception of kids who have allergies and can't eat just anything). The very foods that Mrs. Obama and RFK demonize are preferred by kids, especially picky eaters, neurodivergent kids, and those with eating disorders like ARFID, because they are relatively stable in taste, texture, and appearance. So, we find ourselves in a conundrum that really leads me to one conclusion: sometimes, fed is best. Food moralization doesn't just harm kids with eating disorders or increase the likelihood that they'll develop them; it also invites food rules and rituals borne of class and race privilege. Eating exclusively-plant based or organic food is not an accessible reality to all Americans, and we can argue for making that access a reality without shaming kids and their families for eating food that comes in packages. School mealtimes offer a chance for kids who struggle with eating and body image to try new foods, study school lunch menus, and explore tastes, textures, and flavors of food they may not try otherwise.

Fear of fat is pervasive in the lunchroom; and the combination of the social hierarchy of the lunchbox, earlier onset of dieting and disordered eating, and the influence of parenting, media, and marketing, all play a role. The Bauer survey also found that "Many girls [in the study] discussed how they felt uncomfortable eating in front of the boys in the cafeteria because they feel eating in public makes them look unattractive and do not want to be seen 'stuffing their face.'"[5] This was a popular sentiment at my sixth grade lunch table, so much so that it drove one of my tablemates to anorexia; and the more we encouraged her to eat, the less she did.

A possibility for ending food shame (and, by extension, body shame) is the hopeful result of an "all foods fit" approach. Food shame and anxiety at school haven't always been about what students eat, but *how, how much*, and *when* they eat. Liz Browne, whom I spoke to in Chapter 3 about health, recalls conversations overheard while on lunch duty about kids whose parents "only *let* them eat Annie's mac and cheese," which implies more virtue in the organic option as opposed to other brands like Kraft. Instead of feeding into the narrative that some foods are "better" than others, what if we encouraged students to ask *why* this was the case and how and by whom they were taught that idea? What if we questioned what "better for you" means, and interrogated whether the implication is actually just "this brand is less likely to make you gain weight?"

The nutritional requirements in school meals can also sometimes mean that students throw away the food they don't want. Despite studies finding that there has not been an increase in plate waste in school cafeterias[275] since the implementation of the Obama-era initiatives, schools still waste, on average, 530,000 tons of food per year. Because of these nutritional guidelines, students may be required to take milk or a fruit with their tray, even if they won't eat it. Some schools set up a "donate/share" or "give back" bin for the food they get on their plates that they don't want – a way to offset food waste. But where does it go from there? Is it donated to students, families, or community organizations helping fight food insecurity?

Sugar, You're Going Down

Making an enemy of sugar does not resolve the problems of necessary transparency, consistency, accuracy, and access to nutrition in our school cafeterias and beyond. It does provide, however, a convenient scapegoat to distract from the quality of other foods like meat and dairy; both of which remain heavily marketed in our national political landscape and frozen in the cafeteria kitchen.

But if students are getting the message that sugar (and fat) is bad *from* school, and having it reinforced at home, too, it could encourage the kind of relationship with food that we claim we want to avoid. Because if we are teaching kids that this food is "bad," such restrictive policy and attitude can backfire – leading kids to seek the food out in secret, and in larger quantities than they would have if they didn't feel ashamed to eat it. When we create cultures and cafeterias that confuse kids about food, and even make them afraid to eat, it increases the likelihood that they will engage in furtive eating behaviors – a symptom of binge eating disorder. Aubrey Gordon notes this experience in her first book:

> Every encounter with forbidden foods became a time to load up on them. As I got older, this meant eating contraband foods in secret and hiding foods to eat when I was alone. Shame taught me to overeat and to fetishize food. The more it was withheld, the more tempting it became.[17]

The removal of "unhealthy" snacks and the replacement with low-fat, reduced-fat alternatives may lead to the same levels of reactance, or an increased desire for the "forbidden" foods.[279]

Thirteen years after the launch of *Let's Move!*, Mrs. Obama has launched Plezi Nutrition, a public benefit corporation dedicated to "raising a healthier generation of kids." This is exactly the slogan and goal of the campaign she led as FLOTUS, except now the goal is to sell that promise in stores.[270] The main product is a fruit juice drink, marketed to ages six and up, that "contains 75% less sugar than leading 100% fruit juices." The drink is sweetened with stevia and monk fruit extract, which is a no-calorie sweetener tens of times sweeter than refined sugar, and deemed "generally recognized as safe" (GRAS) by the FDA.[280] Plezi Nutrition, Obama has promised, will "jumpstart a race to the top that will transform the entire food industry."[270]

There it is: her connection to her husband's educational policy, Race to the Top, a policy implemented by President Barack Obama, a program intended to bridge the gap in education for underserved, historically marginalized students. Race to the Top increased educational grants, improved standards and assessment, and improved data and progress monitoring.[281] Using the language of this program, Mrs. Obama's goal to "transform the entire food industry," begins with marketing and consumerism. In her article, Virginia Sole Smith states,

> It's straight up diet culture to tell consumers that their children's health crisis is a problem we can solve with... shopping. Putting the responsibility on parents to "make better choices" has long enabled Big Food to avoid

regulation that would hold them to higher standards in the first place.[270]

And, lest we forget, Mrs. Obama's original campaign worked within these same food industries that she worked with a decade ago to reduce the calories in packaged snacks at schools across America – an effort which, generally, did not totally succeed in making food composition healthier overall. The packaged foods made available at school remained similar in fat and other ways, including fat, sodium, etc. – some retaining their status as ultraprocessed foods. Similarly, the Plezi drinks contain up to five different fruit sugars from fruit concentrate, including monk fruit extract, stevia leaf extract, "natural flavors."[282] While the sugar in fruit is a natural ingredient, it's debatable whether its presence in these drinks makes kids "crave sweets less." The company's goal is to

> give parents a helping hand by offering healthier, great-tasting products that parents can feel good about giving their kids and that kids actually want. Plezi focuses on lowering sugar content and lowering sweetness to help adjust kids' palates to crave less sweetness overall. In addition to reducing the sugar and sweetness, they are adding in nutrients kids need, all with the aim to replace sugary drinks and snacks.

Monkfruit extract, present in some of the Plezi offerings, such as Blueberry Blast and Sour Apple, however, is according to some research up to two hundred times sweeter than table sugar. This, readers should know, is not a call to demonize sugar – but instead, a questioning of the open contradictions of these kinds of initiatives and brands, especially when the goal is to sell a product. The ethos of Plezi, just like with *Let's Move!*, is to "make kids healthier," but does so by putting the onus on parents and profits to do so.

To date, the Plezi brand has donated $1 million to FoodCorps' Nourishing Futures initiative, a campaign that is working toward universal free school meals and nutrition education by 2030.

This cause, aiming to reduce lunch debt (which shouldn't even be a thing), is a worthwhile, systematic change – one that prioritizes feeding kids. Under the Biden administration, Nourishing Futures was "announced in collaboration with the White House Conference on Hunger, Nutrition, and Health," and aims to "Mobilize 1 million supporters for policies that expand access to nourishing school meals; fund food educators; update garden, kitchen, and cafeteria infrastructure; strengthen local supply chains; and, support the food education and school nutrition workforce."[283] Its sponsors, alongside Plezi, include the W.K. Kellogg Foundation, the Newman's Own Foundation, Mars Food (the creators of M&Ms and other chocolate), Orgain Clean Nutrition, Thrive Market, and the Walmart Foundation.[283] The site also has lessons for teachers to implement in classrooms, including one for fifth graders called "Sugar Showdown." The "Sugar Facts" worksheet includes a statement that reads:

"'We need to eat added sugar just like we need to eat fats and protein.' **False.** Although our bodies need sugar to function properly, our bodies can get sugar from eating plants (grains, starches, vegetables, and fruits) and other things in our diet. We don't need to eat any added sugar."[284]

It also introduces the rhetoric of "empty calories," while emphasizing that food is about identity, connection, belonging, and culture elsewhere on the website. If food is about all these things, but we're also saying that added sugar is unnecessary or "bad," then how are students supposed to balance these conflicting truths while enjoying a birthday celebration or fun with friends? This is a setup for confusing, conflicting, and potentially restrictive relationships with food throughout their school experience.

> **Quick Tip**
>
> If your school has policies that ban sugar or specific foods from being sold, brought in, or eaten in class for any reason other than potential allergen exposure – interrogate it; is this policy and its intended purpose rooted in diet culture, or definitions of health born of the thin ideal?

Instead, teaching kids to invite sugar into their meals in moderation creates an effect that suggests to the brain that they are available anytime, and reduces the brain's need to do a "last supper" binge every time they eat a sugary food. If they have permission to eat all foods, moderation about them is more likely. Registered dietitians Karen Ansel and Esther Ellis say that "when kids fill up on sugar-sweetened foods and beverages they have little appetite for healthier foods their growing bodies need, such as fruits, vegetables, whole grains, lean protein, and low-fat dairy." "Pairing sugar with other nutrients like fat, protein and fiber ensures sweetness is met with a side of additional nutrition."[285] It also approaches eating from a place of abundance, rather than restriction; adding nutrient density rather than subtracting and moralizing it has helped me personally on my own journey with food.

While eating food can be social, celebratory, and rewarding, there are many issues with using it as a reward. Extrinsically rewarded food is one way in which eating becomes social control. This is a common practice among teachers, who dole out candy during review games and in exchange for good behavior (which I've been guilty of in my own career). What "food as reward" teaches kids is that they have to "earn their way" to eat something they enjoy. They can only eat if they "deserve" it, and only if the food given to them is handed out by an authority figure. When we juxtapose this with the expectation that they don't eat in your class otherwise, it can also be confusing. The framing of candy and other sweet treats as a reward also confuses student hunger and fullness cues and rewires brain reward circuitry, widening the potential for students to be out of touch with their bodies and eat when not hungry.[286] Using food as a reward may also lead kids with larger bodies to seem more "eager," and feed into the stereotype that they are binge eaters or fixated with eating – increasing teasing from their peers.

"Allowing" students to eat in class or not is also a way that we build compliance and control around food, which can be an issue for a number of reasons; namely, that the multi-period day means some kids eat early and are hungry for the rest of the day, or have a late lunch period and spend their morning with a rumble in their belly that makes them dysregulated and unable to focus. Understandably, having students eat in class can pose a few problems, including food comparison, distraction, and disposal of food waste and packaging. The expectation that students help maintain the classroom and minimize litter so that everyone can learn and listen to their bodies at the same time is a way to build food-positive, body-positive learning spaces.

> **Quick Tip**
>
> *Reconsider the ways that "food as reward" and incentives (even things as small as candy) might be reinforcing a problematic relationship with food. Instead, rewards like class in another part of the building, stickers or fidgets, or unstructured free time.*

In an effort to promote "health," some schools are telling students what they can and cannot bring to school for lunch. Policies that seek to eliminate entire food experiences for students aren't just problematic because they reinforce diet culture – they assume that everyone in the community has the same values, food access, and food prep time.

Dr. Polson, whom you met in Chapter 2, reflected with me on the ways his policies and framing of wellness as a school leader have evolved since he started teaching.

> As a young phys ed teacher, I was on the wellness policy development [committee] for the district in 2003–2004, and that was a big nutrition kick, ramped up [professional development] hours, more understanding of physical activity, and one focus was about children and sugar,

he said.

> One thing they had at my first school was a sugar policy. When I came to my new district, they had a wellness policy, but it didn't include that; so that was something I was vocal and adamant about. For the longest time, I was the only school adhering to that strictly because I thought it was something that was important.

Today, he said, policies look a little different at Northern Parkway Elementary – for example, if teachers host a pizza party, it takes the place of lunch. But as of 2022, sugar is back on the table at classroom celebrations, teacher functions, and "publishing parties" where students showcase their writing. And though Northern Parkway's breakfast hours exist officially between 7:45 and 8:30, kids can get breakfast all day before lunch at 11 if they are hungry; thanks to the school's lead cook, Miss Erica.

> She treats this kitchen like her home kitchen. She's making food for over six hundred children, but you'd think she's making it for a group of sixty, sixteen or six. She's the one who interrupted the rule without me even knowing, until lunch is served. So our policies have been interrupted with and without my awareness,

he says, based on the needs of his students and the intuition and leadership of all who make wellness possible at school.

Polson mentioned that a large consideration he made when thinking about food and celebrations at school was through the lens of culturally relevant, responsive, and (not yet) sustaining pedagogy,[287] citing that he feared that bringing in food from different ethnicities and cultures became synonymous with cultural relevance. While food is culture, socialization, love, and community – the presence of food is not an effective change needed to make education more holistically equitable for kids or teachers. "Doing diversity" and making people *feel* seen are not the same as ensuring that they *are* seen.

Dr. Polson said many teachers struggled with the moratorium on sweets in the classroom and even at faculty celebrations. But Polson isn't alone in this thinking. The early 2000s were the time of "the threat of fat kids is worse than terrorism" – remember? How could any teacher, no matter where they were in their career, not be alarmed if they were taught to perceive that the situation was indeed that dire? "I was adamant that when children are with us [at school], we need to make sure they have all the 'right foods' around and with them." His school is a "fresh food and vegetable school," a success he attributes to government programs like the USDA guidelines – "the kids love trying new things," he says, "and it's great because they find out things they really love, and things they try and say "that's nasty, I don't think I want to eat that again!" which is totally fine!" Crafting school food attitudes that ensure that all foods are an option and that students and teachers have the opportunity to regulate what, when, and how much they eat allows them to follow their body throughout the school day and become better learners. In general across America, kids are now eating 16 percent more vegetables and 23 percent more fruit at lunch – which the USDA attributes to the Hunger Free Healthy Kids Act. This is not to suggest that that's "better" than eating Doritos, but emphasizes that kids having wide varieties of *choice* about what to eat is critical to food justice and school equity.[288]

"As a principal and as a teacher, I have a responsibility to lead-learn," he said, citing the concept from Roland S. Barth. "As a model and as a learner, I can say I thought I knew a thing, and now I know more about a thing and I get to share that with you," "It's okay to think one thing and then as you learn differently, you behave differently."

Dr. Taylor Arnold, the kid nutritionist, outlines her thoughts about low/no sugar policies in an Instagram post: "Low sugar convenience foods like granola bars are often more expensive," she says in an Instagram video. The cost of these convenience foods may be prohibitive to single moms and dads packing lunch in a hurry, who have only one source of income. Arnold adds, "I hate the idea of teachers having to confiscate food from a child if it's not a safety concern." She also says that low/no sugar policies "limit the variety parents can send to school with their kids, which is REALLY hard for kids with already limited diets due to ARFID, autism, ADHD and allergies."

The one study done in 1973 by allergist Benjamin Feingold, on one kid, has become the cultural basis for the myth of the "sugar high."[289] Feingold didn't advocate for eliminating sugar, but he suggested that parents would be best served by avoiding additives.[290] Because sugar comes from natural and refined sources, Feingold lumped sugar in with "additives." Since then, studies have tested the theory of the "sugar high," and have not found anything conclusive.

> We don't have any evidence that low sugar policies actually help kids in school, but rather they may hurt kids. These policies make lunch much more difficult for kids with food allergies and pediatric feeding disorders, and low income families. These restrictions can also make establishing healthy relationships with food more difficult for many families,

said Dr. Taylor Arnold in an Instagram post.[291]

School-sanctioned sugar elimination also exposes class, cultural, and other differences in ways that are not celebratory or even, at best, neutral. What food policing and inequity then manifests is parent blame and shame. Parents who send their kids to school with Oreos because their kid enjoys them (or because it's one of their safe foods) are seen as "better" parents than the moms who pack $42 Omie boxes and cucumbers cut into fun shapes.[223] Treating foods like contraband and treating them as the "wrong" foods to eat creates an environment of shame and othering that brings about trauma. When we send kids home with notes about the "forbidden" foods they brought to school that day, asking nicely to please not send him with chips again, we attempt to shape the behavior of parents – and their kids – through shame that is often racialized, gendered, ableist, and classist as well as fatphobic. Psyche Williams-Forson puts it this way: "It is far more convenient and easier to reduce the whole of African American foodstuffs to that which is simple, neat and compact, no matter how erroneous." She says that the danger of the narratives around Black, working class, poor, and I would add, fat, bodies and how they eat is harmful because of "what people become in their own minds, not to mention the minds of others. This is what leads to policies, decisions, and ways of interacting with people that cast them as inferior and incapable."[227]

Now, we have discourse around "good sugar" and "bad sugar," and a host of ways that we blame sugar for everything from diabetes to ADHD. Ansel and Ellis posit that at parties and celebrations, actually, kids are more excited and amped up about the social interactions they're having with their friends, not necessarily the cake and pizza they're eating.[289] So maybe the solution isn't banning sugary foods: it's more unstructured social and play time and joy.

Where'd All the Time Go?

On average, schools give students 25–30 minutes for lunch, and the length of a "class period" in secondary school is typically about 40 minutes; that length of time includes periods designated for lunch.[221] As it stands, fewer than half of schools meet the CDC recommendation of 20 minutes of seat time in the cafeteria.[292] According to a survey by the School Nutrition Association, students also must use that time to use the restroom, walk to the cafeteria, survey their lunch options, and stand in line – all of which does not add up to enough seat time to complete a meal thoughtfully in most cases.[293] This is not good for their digestion or their habituation around food; eating food too fast because you're in a rush is the antithesis of mindful eating. I've had students whose lunch period is right before my class bring their entire meal to class, because they prioritized getting to play basketball with friends or sit and decompress after a difficult exam. Allowing them the flexibility that our schedules do not is part of humanizing teaching and helping students listen to their bodies. The SNA states that federal regulations state that "schools must offer lunches between 10:00 am and 2:00 pm." These regulations also encourage schools to "provide sufficient lunch periods that are long enough to give all students adequate time to be served and to eat their lunches." Schools may request exemptions from these times from their state education agencies.[221]

At Dr. Polson's school, they do "fitness Fridays," during which movement is made part of the morning meeting. One STEAM teacher is even yoga certified, and includes mindfulness and asanas (poses) into the movement routines.

Movement is critical – sometimes you have to shut it down and just go outside and play, and come back and get to [learning]. I do believe in sustained learning, and I believe they also need to know what it means to interrupt that so they can learn for longer.

As of 2023, policymakers in states like Maine, Rhode Island, South Carolina and Vermont are all considering legislation that would establish a minimum number of minutes for lunch periods.[293] This comes as a positive and welcome change amidst the pandemic, where some schools shortened periods to 15 minutes to maintain social distancing and limit the spread of illness, offering more "grab and go" options as well.

Having to throw their lunch out because of insufficient eating time is also a huge source of food waste in the cafeteria, which costs America over $1.2 billion per year. More time to eat mindfully, assess their hunger and fullness cues, and socially reset with peers means more nutrition, and allows for better cognitive functioning and the ability to learn for the rest of their day[292, 294]; lunchtime should be a time for students to relax, breathe, slow down, and de-stress from morning classes.[292] Current research from the CDC focuses on the idea that more time to eat means more time to consume fruits and vegetables (as opposed to prepackaged foods), which is, of course, not inherently bad – but still prioritizes some foods over others.[294] For example, the CDC says kids with more time for lunch are "more likely to select a fruit," which amounts to moralizing their choices and suggests that some food choices are arbitrarily superior to others.[293] We create a moral quagmire by making both whole and prepackaged foods available in the first place – why are we praising kids for choosing fruits and veggies, knowing that we serve chips, cookies, and even ice cream – if we're going to admonish them for it, both implicitly and explicitly? It puts kids in a position to socially assess one another about their food choices, manufacturing body prejudice and stereotypes around food and what their choices supposedly "mean" about them. Peers are more likely to ridicule, stereotype, and blame kids in larger bodies who choose the cookies and chips, for example, for the way their bodies look; but if they choose the apple, that doesn't fit the fatphobic narrative we've built around them – and all of that is a function of anti-fat bias.

What if we centered our attention not on what kids consume if we give them more time, but the fact that they get to listen to their body, honor their hunger and fullness, choose foods they like to eat, and take a much-needed break in ways that feel accessible and positive to them? Recess and lunch are one part of the day where students have a choice in what they do – and empowering them to make decisions is a fundamental part of making their learning more human. Several examples of longer lunches and their positive effects include Arundel High School in Maryland, which gives students a 50-minute lunch period. This allows them to get lunch, eat lunch, catch up with teachers, and socialize. Students reported appreciation for the extra time to catch up with friends and get extra help they need from teachers. The school's principal, Sharon Stratton, said this change not only allows students to form a community but also can lead to less stress and higher grades.[295] The article title, "Longer Lunch, More Options" points to exactly what students need: increased choice about how to spend their time, how to move their bodies, and what to eat without moralizing or shame.

There are many approaches to scheduling lunch that work – and plenty that don't. For all three years I was in middle school, I had fourth period lunch on my schedule. Fourth period lunch began at 9:40 am, which was hardly lunch time at all. As I started running fall cross country and spring track, the time of day I ate lunch became even more futile. For many students who participate in sports, this is the case. But even if they don't, eating lunch two hours into the school day and not getting an opportunity to take a break or eat again until they're home (assuming they have food at

> **Quick Tip**
>
> *Build classroom policy with students for eating during class time; do not ask students to justify why they want or need to eat during class. Instead, negotiate expectations that include keeping the classroom clean, minimizing distractions, and minding the allergies and sensory needs of those around them.*

home) is unhelpful at best, and unhealthy at worst. When students emerge from unstructured time ready to learn, it sets them up for success – but not if they eat too soon or too late and spend the day focused on hunger.

Recess or break time is an important part of the school day for kids of all ages. I always valued the unstructured time of being able to go outside during elementary school, even if it was just to read a book under a shady tree – because I could choose what to do during that precious half hour outside. Though it's mostly seen in elementary schools, recess is increasingly present in secondary schools as well. Ryan Nguyen, a high school sophomore, advocates for recess in a *Scholastic Choices* article:

> We need a break! Ask a teen about their day, and they'll likely give you a long list of classes, extracurricular activities, and schoolwork. I've witnessed so much anxiety related to these hectic schedules: students pulling the fire alarm during midyear exams, kids sobbing in class, and even a girl fainting during a test. With today's intense pressure to succeed, many teens are pushed to take on too many responsibilities at the expense of sleep, exercise, and free time. [296]

Research shows that brain breaks can boost motivation and improve a student's mood. [297] Recess doesn't have to emphasize movement and physical activity in order to benefit everyone. In an article for CommonLit, author Kaylin Oliver states:

> The key to an ideal recess is a balance of options. "Choice is the biggest thing that comes to mind, balancing the needs of introverts and the needs of extroverts," said Kenan Kerr, a former North Carolina teacher and facilitator. [298]

Even for kids who do want to think about academics during their free time, having the agency to go ask a teacher a question privately or in a small group can alleviate a lot of the pressure they feel about their work. The impact lies in the option and having access to the time to self-advocate.

For kids in larger bodies, recess offers them a chance to make the choice to participate in movement how they want to, make new friends, or, like me, read a book and just be outside. Due to the nature of unstructured play that happens at recess, though, fat kids may find themselves subject to teasing and bullying that is expressly about their weight. The playground is a place where anti-fat harm has the potential to increase, especially in the elementary setting where multiple classes are in the same space. While increasing movement is often a stated goal for "preventing obesity," the reality is that fat kids who engage in movement are often still laughed at by their peers. So even when they're doing the "good" and "right" thing (according to diet culture), they are subject to ridicule – they can't win.

This points to the need for more watchful supervision of play, higher expectations of inclusion that specifically mention weight bias and how to prevent it. The need for body bias training among those who supervise the cafeteria and the playground is important, because weight-based bullying can happen at the hand of "trusted" adults, too. Remember my example from Chapter 1, about my after-school care provider? "At least he's moving/playing/trying to be 'good!'" aren't helpful responses to weight-based teasing encountered by fat kids just trying to feel included in a game of kickball or freeze tag – it only fossilizes the notion that the only "good" way to be in a fat body is by performing athleticism or "trying" to become different (thinner). It isn't just in our curriculum, it's in our comments, and what we allow to happen and how we allow children in larger bodies to feel about themselves. Overhearing jokes about size, weight or clothing from adults, talking about people's food choices, or even self-directed body shame can, and does, influence our kids.[299] Recess presents schools with a unique opportunity to shape school culture; if kids do opt for physical activity, no matter what body they show up in, setting an expectation that promotes positivity and inclusion makes body shaming unthinkable and instead promotes having

> **Quick Tip**
>
> Advocate for adequate recess and recreation time for students in all grades, and set inclusive standards and expectations for play during those unstructured times in your school.

fun and cheering each other on over cutthroat competition and winning. This kind of culture building has the potential to make recess, and participation in activities that go on during unstructured time, as a positive experience for everyone, not just the most athletically inclined kids on the court or field.

In Ogden City School District in Utah, staff reward students with more extended lunch periods if they reduce their lateness to class and keep up with grades. Since the program began, the principal at the high school notes that student lateness has been reduced by half.[300] While this practice offers incentive to do well in school, it tells students that they have to *earn* time to exist as themselves instead of it just being built into their day. On the other side of the same coin is the practice of withholding recess for behavior or missed work, and the concept of "lunch detention." Such practices often punish students of color and students with disabilities more disproportionately, and don't address the root of the problem. Policies that do this signal to kids that free movement and bodily autonomy, which help them regulate, are a privilege. It falls under the same category as incentivizing classroom behavior and academic achievement with food; we cannot make a commodity out of things our students need to function. Isolating students is, again, the opposite of prosocial behavior; schools should opt for lunch groups and restorative opportunities instead of taking away the little time students have to relax and recharge.

Currently, no federal efforts to protect kids from recess withholding exist in the United States. A survey from 2022 indicates that up to 86 percent of American teachers have withheld or decreased recess or recreational time from students in response to behavioral or academic issues.[301] However, several states such as California and Illinois have passed legislation to define recess and prevent schools from forcing students to sit out for disciplinary reasons. Illinois regulations make an exception only when a student's participation is an immediate safety threat.[302] Other states, like New Jersey and Rhode Island, more permissively allow recess withholding as a practice. New Jersey's law indicates that teachers cannot withhold recess more than twice a week, and only if the student violates district codes of conduct.[301] Many districts make recess or lunch detention part of their explicitly stated disciplinary procedure as a "possible or mandatory consequence" for different student behaviors. And even when districts adopt policies against recess withholding, research shows that statewide laws, not district policies, make the biggest difference in protecting kids' right to play.[301]

RUN IT BACK – Reflecting on Your Practice

♦ *What might an "all foods fit" approach look like at my school?*

♦ *What is my role in helping my school create or maintain an approach that is food and body neutral (at a minimum) and/ or positive (at best)?*

♦ *How can our school improve its relationship to food in our community? Who do we need to invite to these conversations?*

♦ *Does my school give kids (and teachers) enough time to eat during their lunch period? Do we allow them opportunities to nourish their bodies outside the cafeteria?*

♦ *Do I believe recess and "break times" are a privilege, or a right? How can I honor and value the need to reset as a part of my students' education?*

7

School's Out

Fighting Weight Stigma in Extracurricular Activity

After-school activities that fuel kids' passions help them feel a sense of greater belonging, hope, and community with their school environment. School is more than a learning environment, and the social component of school – namely extracurriculars like sports, clubs, drama, music, and art programs – have the power to give kids a space to pursue their interests and passions beyond the basic curriculum.

Everyone emphasizes the "well-rounded" student who can put a million clubs, teams, and accolades on their college resume. I always related more to the Athenians of ancient Greece (book smart) than the Spartans (the combat warriors), even when I was a two-season athlete. "At least she's smart," is the new "at least you have a nice *face*," that bestows pity upon the fat kid for not conforming, as a way of saying "your body is unacceptable to us, but at least you can be useful or redeemed for something else." This is anti-fat bias, plain, and simple. Doing the work of ensuring that kids have safe, non-academic spaces to go to that are free of weight stigma is especially important for fat kids.[303]

DOI: 10.4324/9781003534143-9

A lot of fat kids' initial assessment of their value is that they're never going to be good enough until they're thin. But if they had something that created supports or protective factors, it can have a huge positive impact for fat-related trauma experience. Having a place where their body wasn't the main focus, where they could just exist – it wouldn't even have to be a fat-positive space, it could just be a neutral space – it could get in the way of building a trauma response,

said Kayla Stansberry, a Virginia-based therapist.

When fat kids are told all day that the desks they try to sit in can't hold them, the lunch they prefer is bad for them, or the body they live in is a source of disgust projected onto them by others – after-school activities become more than a passion; they can be a lifeline. Kayla told me that "Being involved in something outside of yourself is a great resource in building community, strengthening relationships with others, and teaches people how to do that outside of areas of 'ease.'" But these escapes from the fatphobia embedded into academia are not guaranteed to end, and almost always do not end, at the bell. Stansberry said, "For larger bodied kids, it's hard not to see it through the lens of it not [always] being good." For example, "making weight" on the wrestling team, being cut from the cheerleading squad, or being typecast as the sidekick or the leading role in the school play. Kayla continued, "If it's a safe environment, it lets kids know that it's okay to exist in their bodies in a safe way." Let's begin there.

You Can't Stop the Beat(s)

Who knew the 1980s would produce one of the most fat-positive (albeit still problematic) musicals our culture can name? *Hairspray*, written in the 1980s but set in the 1960s, features Tracy Turnblad and her mom, Edna, both of whom are fat and, this means, of course, not the "ideal" girl. You've probably seen it – and if you haven't, at least watch the 2007 remake starring Nikki Blonsky and Zac Efron.

In her essay about it for *The Other F Word*, Amy Spalding reflects on Tracy Turnblad and her importance as a cultural heroine who fights for her place as the best dancer on her favorite after-school special and to end broadcasting segregation in Baltimore. Spalding states "Since I was young, theater had space for characters of all colors in ways I wasn't necessarily seeing in mainstream film or television."[32] Much of the plot of *Hairspray* is about being fat – but, Spalding says, "it didn't seem to bring us any closer to better representations of fat people in the media."[32] I've seen this play performed in high schools I've worked in. What about plays that aren't about being fat – and the messages we send to fat kids in theater programs when we put them in the ensemble, or even backstage, to be unseen and unheard because they don't "fit"? In theater, the term typecasting is often used to gatekeep who can and cannot play a role. "Casting is a form of communication," says Abby Rose Morris, the host of the *More than Tracy Turnblad* podcast. "When you cast fat students in the ensemble, instead of lead roles, especially lead roles where there is a romantic storyline, you are telling them that they can't be that because it wouldn't be believable," she said.

> But you tell them, hey, you can be the mom, and then we layer assumptions about how the mom became fat (she had kids, etc.) and ironically miss the point that she must be desirable in some way if she's a mom and she's married.

In plays like *Hairspray*, Tracy should be played by a fat person (as opposed to a thin person in a fat suit, which makes the fat body *become* the joke), and a character like Motormouth Maybelle must be played by a Black woman. But under certain conditions, typecasting can be exclusionary for the wrong reasons. Why can't Sandy be fat in *Grease or* Mary Swanson be fat in *Middletown*?

In her interview for *Burnt Toast*, actress Katy Geraghty says, "We need to keep telling these kids that just because no one like you has played it doesn't mean no one ever will." Just hiring fat actors to play in roles isn't enough, especially in smaller scale, kid-facing theater programs:

> If you're going to be diverse in casting, you also have to think about it through the whole show. Like don't just think about the fact that yes, we did the job and they're going to be on stage. That might also mean you need two more feet on each step because you have some bigger bodied people on stage.[304]

Art programming needs so much more funding in general, but the lack of availability might mean that kids must "choose" (without much choice) theater programs that are anti-fat and not safe for them to be part of. Having ongoing conversations about things like costume deadlines (which may need an extension for kids who need extended sizing) or scripts that feature anti-fat jokes and humor or turn fat characters into punchlines – which, even in the 2007 remake, was an issue in Hairspray – can help create more inclusive spaces for fat characters that uplift their experiences in theater beyond tokenistic representation and slapstick bullying. Katy Geraghty presents a list of questions for fat theater kids and their parents to consider when looking at a program: "Are they [fat people] on stage at all? Are they in front? Are they the ones that look happy to be there?"[304]

Moreover, in the presence of the "controversial," something called "table work" often happens in theater. Table work is the act of collectively understanding a play's social, political, contemporary, or identity-based context together as a cast. Table work is a necessary step of bringing a script to life, and should happen every time, especially in spaces where learning is happening, such as schools. Artists create art to imitate life, and life has not historically been free of oppression for everyone. Having high school and even middle school casts understand the ways that certain humor has not aged, specifically racist, sexist, xenophobic, or fatphobic humor, can help all cast members raise consciousness about oppression beyond the script and the score. It can also mean that the cast members who are parts of the community that are represented problematically in the script don't have to shoulder the pain of harmful, often unchangeable original scripts, alone. Making cast members aware that for some, being the butt of a cruel joke isn't just a script – it's life. Even in secondary schooling contexts, changing the script to weed out the offensive stuff is tricky, and can be entirely illegal due to licensing. But that's worth talking about: if someone in the cast or the audience will face harm because of this play, should this play be something we perform? Starting the process of casting and rehearsing even a week earlier than scheduled so that actors can do this important work can be critical to school-based theater programs, and offer educational opportunities. And in the event that a school play is a period piece – like *Hairspray* or *Newsies* (both plays with fat characters!) Theater educators may invite teachers from subjects other than drama (English, PE, social studies) to have conversations with students about the script, the context, and the historiography of the play. It's a great opportunity for theater to become a community effort, rather than just something that "theater kids" do.

"It's more important in educational theater settings to give kids an experience that will make them want to keep doing theater, rather than being exactly to the letter of the script all the time," Abby Rose Morris said. "Theater is psychology, embodiment, and so much more, but primarily, theater is empathy…and making it believable is less important than allowing students to learn a lot, feel valued, explore, and have fun." Abby says that when she was younger, she focused a lot on getting the show "perfect," and expecting it to be Broadway quality – she wanted the stereotypical intensity of a theater production, complete with screaming directors and long hours – but as an adult, she looks back and says that those were not the experiences that shaped her love of theater and acting at all.

When I was in summer camp before middle school, we did *Mary Poppins* – and they thought I was talented enough to play the role of Mary Poppins – and I really remember that. That was one of the last times for me that my experience in theater was about just enjoying a role.

And, in those auditoriums and theater seats, fat bodies still don't always fit, either. So what good is representation, or a play about representation, if the world that play exists in hasn't evolved beyond fiction and the catchy show tunes it produces? Just like in airplanes, more seats equal more money, which is ultimately what motivates theater seating to be built so small. Katy Geraghty again, says that seating that is not inclusive is like "saying 'you don't even deserve to watch [a play], let alone be in it.'"[304]

The Eye of the Tiger: Wrestling with Weight Stigma in Sports

Like plays and musicals, sports are a performing art of their own in a way. As I previously mentioned, I was an athlete two seasons a year from seventh to tenth grade. I ran cross country in the fall and track in the spring. Some of my teammates ran winter track and didn't take the season off, but I just couldn't commit and knew it was best to rest.

> The way we approach sports in schools is not good for students' mental health, and a lot of it is because of what the adults (coaches, parents, trainers) do. They are taught to value themselves and their peers because of a rigid expectation – everything is about winning, hard work, scholarships. Sports can teach great skills, but the way they are taught is problematic,

said Kayla Stansberry, also known on Instagram as @fatpositivetherapist.

How many kids aren't engaging in extracurricular activities that involve movement because of their bodies? "Having teams available that are just about fun and movement can be a game changer [for fat kids]," said Kayla. Paying teachers as club advisors who can host intramural teams, or even partnering with free or nonprofit intramural teams to build after-school connections can help kids foster a sense of belonging that isn't about rigid, serious competition and less likely to get them typecast for a role on the field or on the court – if not sidelined or pity-rostered onto a school-sponsored team, just to be declared the "manager" or spend the season on the bench.

Similar to how fat kids have always been erased from public life through shaming and food policing, politicians are currently trying to erase trans kids from things like intramural and team sports. I mention this because the forces that perpetuate anti-trans bias and anti-fat bias are one and the same. Under the Biden administration, the federal government attempted to widen the implementation of Title IX to include trans students, so that they could participate equally in all aspects of public life, particularly related to their education. As a response, the cry to "protect women and girls in sports" has taken hold among more conservative circles, from local county municipalities to the White House. In my birth county of Nassau, New York, county executive Bruce Blakeman implemented a ban on trans athletes playing at any county facilities. In 2024, the Long Island Roller Rebels, along with the NYCLU, sued the county over the decision, and won the first of a series of lawsuits against Blakeman and his ban.[305] The county facilities, however, host mostly intramural teams, including those played on by kids. As stated in previous chapters, sports at such a young age aren't really about winning – they're about building empathy, teamwork, sportsmanship, and skills – and when adults take those opportunities away from trans kids and fat kids alike, the message is clear: you don't belong. The following year, a state legislature bill (S460) was introduced in an effort to ban trans kids from participating in sports as the gender they identify as. Conservative State Senator Steven Rhoads, who hails from Nassau County's fifth senate district (my home district), sponsored the bill.[306]

Even more important to this dynamic is that trans people, especially adolescents, are more susceptible to body dysmorphia and body hate – dysphoria and dysmorphia tend to go hand in hand. As we learned in Chapter 1, trans kids face a more frequent onslaught of weight-based bullying. But important to note in terms of athletics is that trans people have a higher incidence of eating disorders, too. Transgender individuals, as a whole, "are at increased risk for developing ED/DEB [eating disorder/disordered eating behaviors] due to a number of factors including: gender dysphoria, minority stress, the desire to pass, and barriers to gender affirming care."[307] Couple that with the body struggles of adolescence, and eating disorders become even more likely. From there, excluding transgender children from activities they love is only going to lead to more isolation, poorer mental health outcomes, and an increased need for eating disorder treatment. If these same politicians who worry about "protecting girls in sports," where is their energy when it comes to fighting eating disorders among cisgender women and girl athletes? How are they funding girls' athletic endeavors compared to those of boys in their local municipalities? And why, if their worry is "making competition fair," are they targeting athletes – children – for whom having fun matters more than competing to win? And how are we supposed to trust that those in power, with serial histories of violating the rights of women and admitting it, care about "protecting" women and girls in sports, or anywhere for that matter?

In her interview for *Burnt Toast*, Frankie de la Cretaz, a journalist and sports writer, says that

> legislation now exists in over half the states because sports were the places where they could make trans people, and trans women in particular, seem threatening. They could couch it in language around fairness, and advantage, and the real marginalization that cis women, and women in general, have faced over time. So sports became the acceptable place for prejudice and discrimination to happen. But the thing is, once you make trans people or any group of people a threat in one arena, it becomes much easier to make them a threat in other parts of life.[148]

Quick Tip

Advocate for equal access and treatment of fat, BIPOC, girl, and trans athletes at your school, so everyone can play. Prioritize things like teamwork, community building, sportsmanship and joy.

In previous chapters, we've discussed how the same exact sentiments have played out on Black bodies. Black people were, and still are, framed as threatening, menacing, out of control, and both subhuman and superhuman at the same time. The formula is the same here: create a problem, blame an entire group, make people afraid of that group, and disappear that group from public life unless they have "separate but equal" access. What we know from this history is that separate, however, is never equal.

To make matters worse, the White House has also chimed in with executive orders that target transgender athletes in these spaces. The executive orders signed in February of 2025 defines gender narrowly and along a binary, stating things such as rising to meet Congress' existing demand for "equal athletic opportunity for members of both sexes" and stripping federal funding away from any institutions "that deny female students an equal opportunity to participate in sports and athletic events by requiring them, in the women's category, to compete with or against or to appear unclothed before males."[308] These kinds of remarks from public officials don't make any women safer or competition more fair; they subject women to more violence, more oppression, and deeper exclusion – especially those who fail to meet the visual standards of whatever they decide a woman is. We've seen these lessons before, played out in the public disparaging of women like South African runner Caster Semenya, and most recently, Algerian boxer Imane Khelif. Both these women have been juxtaposed with the term "DSD," or differences in sexual development, largely based on complaints from women they bested in races or competitions.[309] After her Olympic win, known public figures like J. K. Rowling called her identity as a woman into question.[310] In this case, the IOC recognized that Khelief "was born a woman, registered as a woman, and her passport indicates that she is a woman," and maintained that her medical records are otherwise private information.[311] Still, people speculated or claimed to have seen reports that verify that she is a man or is intersex. In her home country of Algeria and in many places in the world that are even more unsafe for trans people than the United States, false rumors like this can put women in real danger.[312] Frankie de la Cretaz calls policy moves like this "gateway legislation," because it paves the way for policymakers "to pass more extreme anti-trans legislation against healthcare and education."[148]

In some roles where it can be beneficial to the team dynamic to be in a bigger body, body dysmorphia and fat shaming are still rampant. For example, linemen on the football team.

We, as a culture, have ideas about who sports are for: thin people. Which kinds of bodies can be good at sports: thin bodies. We continue to exclude fat people from narratives about sports, despite the fact that fat people are participating, have participated, and are often excelling at all levels of sport.[148]

According to an article for *The Washington Post*, "Fat-shaming has long been associated with the position, and it can be especially cruel in the formative years of teenagers who are aggressively adding body mass in pursuit of college scholarships."[313] With this expectation to be "big" follows the double pressure to be large, but lean – and causes many players in these positions on the field to be the butt end of jokes about their size and weight. The article states:

Many young offensive linemen are racing to add as much weight as possible, which has led some teams to emphasize nutrition and education. At St. John's in Washington, where the offensive linemen range between 280 and 310 pounds, the players' diets are monitored, and they are encouraged to compose food journals. No target weights are set, according to St. John's director of performance training Matt Smith, who also said the team has installed preventive measures to avoid fat shaming.[313]

The purpose of the food journal is to make sure that players don't become "too fat," even though they are running practices and exercising sometimes multiple times a day. The risk of gaining weight in the short period of time that these players do is developing health problems later in life, such as metabolic syndrome and heart issues – but coaches can facilitate food journaling without the weight stigma. De la Cretaz and Sole Smith discuss it in their podcast episode, saying

How often do you see a lineman being the face of a team or the face on the Gatorade bottle? That spotlight goes to the quarterback or the running back or the wide receiver. Their contracts with the NFL are also worth more than lineman contracts. And linemen are much likely to play a much shorter time, and to deal with head injuries later in life. So they might actually need the money more. And that running back doesn't score without the lineman blocking and creating a hole for him to run through. The quarterback doesn't have time to complete the pass if the linemen don't do their job.[148]

In the case of athletes like football linemen, or other larger body-focused sports like rugby, however, a kind of tokenism sets in when it comes to talking about fat players. These positions are useful to the team for things like blocking, so the thinner, more "fit" players in positions like the fullback can score, and outside those moments, are the butt of "playful" jokes among teammates, coaching staff, and peers. When these dynamics take hold on sports teams, a rhetoric of "Wow, even a fat person can be good at this!" rather than just getting respect for the job they do on the field, court, track, or pitch. There is an exceptionalism about it that says "they're a good athlete, despite being fat," instead of just "they're a good athlete, period."[148] Similar to theater, it is a form of typecasting. In some cases, parents of fat kids may just be glad that their kid is being active, being included, or being celebrated for what their body can do – but this can quickly become a kind of backhanded compliment wherever diet culture is present.

> **Quick Tip**
>
> *Before "typecasting" athletes into specific roles on a team based on their weight, size, or appearance, challenge and invite them to try out for different positions on the team. Ask them what their interests are or what they'd like to try. (I was tall enough and could have easily also competed in high jump, for example!) Work with athletes to set guidelines for safe training toward those goals.*

The sport I loved for a brief period of time was one in which, for the most part, my biggest competitor was myself. I didn't love the exposure brought on by track and field, where it was obvious and pretty embarrassing to come in last. Mostly, I ran cross country and track because team sports were something I was too neurodivergent and not coordinated enough to play. Running had only one objective – go, as quickly as possible (track) or as steadily paced as possible (cross country) and breathe regularly. Almost instantly after joining, my coach recruited me for shot put because of my broad shoulders, height, and medium (not skinny, but not "fat" at the time) build.

In a lot of cases, we all sort of circulated the idea that the lighter you are, the faster you go. My compensatory relationship with food likely began here.

For some of my teammates who developed the female athlete triad, it was worse. Being their own biggest competitor was extreme and even potentially dangerous. The female athlete triad is "defined by three concerns: disordered eating, amenorrhea (complete loss of menstrual period) and osteoporosis (loss of bone density)." This phenomenon also happens often in aesthetic sports such as gymnastics, figure skating, or dance.[314] Gabby Guzdek, a former athlete and student at Wesleyan University, says in her article:

> Female athletes are exposed to a unique risk of falling victim to disordered eating behaviors and health issues such as female athlete triad because sports settings are the perfect storm of diet culture messages, gender issues, team culture and athletic performance goals.[314]

Any athlete, coach, or even just avid spectator will tell you that team culture is a function of coaching. I had two teammates who would, quite literally, go back to the coach and rat people out if they did their perimeter run (a pack run where we had to run the perimeter of the entire campus a prescribed number of times as per our coach) by going inside the backstops on the baseball and softball fields instead of outside to cut the distance shorter. There was a sense that someone was always watching, and a coach might make you run it again if you cut the distance even just few meters, instead of telling my teammates to mind their own business and let us feel it in our own individual PR times if we chose to cut corners. So, our bodies weren't only being watched by adults who hoped to help us place in races; they were being monitored by other members of the team.

Being aware of your body because of how it's being judged means that your body isn't yours anymore – it's open for commentary, potentially being sexualized. Especially as girls get older, their body image remains so much of how their bodies are perceived by others,

said Kayla Stansberry. In sports like track and cross country there were ways to "win" the meet if you had the most runners place or a long list of pretty good finishing times, but overall, nobody ever asked or cared if we "won." They took their individual times home with them and used that to get better, stronger, and faster.

Coaches create the space for players to be great; but they can also create the space for players to develop habits that are centered in diet culture and misinformation. Wrestler Lane Shaffer, who wrote an article about his experience being a high school wrestler with an eating disorder, wrote about his experience for *Oregon Live*. "An average person may aim to lose 12 pounds over a month or year. For a competitive wrestler, that's a one-day job. Put on a sweatsuit, do a few hours of cardio and stop eating for a day."[315] "This short term weight loss is physically and psychologically harmful," he continues in the article. "The restriction of food before weigh-ins and the resulting binges disrupt athletes' relationship with food and mirror symptoms of bulimia, an eating disorder characterized by binge eating followed by self-induced vomiting, obsessive dieting or extreme exercise." The reason for weight cycling behavior, Shaffer says, is to compete in a lower weight class, where they may have a better chance of winning.

> **Quick Tip**
>
> *Coaches can host regular pre-season, mid-season, and post-season team meetings to discuss and educate athletes about safe athletic practices, weight modulation, and body image. If you're an athletic director, you can make this a standard practice or requirement of all coaches, regardless of sport, gender, team composition, competition level or age group.*

Many wrestling programs have put in stopgaps to prevent wrestlers from dropping too much weight in order to compete, and in 2021, the NFHS wrote an article addressing its harmful effects especially on young bodies who are still physically developing.

> One-third of high school wrestlers have reported engaging in cyclic weight-control practices more than 10 times per season. Weight cycling or weight cutting practices usually involve one of three methods: 1) decreasing caloric intake, 2) increasing exercise or 3) artificial methods of dehydration. Oftentimes the competitors will employ two or more of these practices simultaneously.[316]

To date, there are no universal standards to prevent harmful weight cycling behaviors in wrestling that I could locate, but the reissue of the 2022–23 NFHS Wrestling Rules (Rule 1, Section 5, Articles 1–3) "outline the process for discouraging excessive weight loss and establishing a safe minimum weight which involves the wrestler, parents/guardians, appropriate healthcare professional and coach." "Discouraging" excessive or rapid weight loss isn't a safeguard against disordered eating or eating disorders; it must be prevented, with school or district-wide policies rooted in child development at the front. As the captain of his wrestling team at McDaniel High School in Portland, Oregon, Shaffer noted that "each wrestler is given a minimum weight that they can drop to, based on their body fat percentage, and is only allowed to lose 1.5% of their weight per week." While this is a guardrail, giving kids who are already predisposed to eating disorders, like Lane, a "minimum weight" may serve for them as an aspiration rather than a safety net. And who's checking?[315]

The NCAA has created rules and safeguards against "cutting weight" as well, as a result of studies that elaborated on the physiological effect of rapid weight cycling not just on wrestler performance during matches, but overall health. These include "a reduction in anaerobic work performance within matches; depleted muscle glycogen levels;

Quick Tip

Certified nurses, dietitians, or athletic trainers who can identify and troubleshoot eating disordered behavior should be accessible to every athlete, coach, and family in schools with sports programming.

reduction in lean body mass; an increase in depression and fatigue."[315]

> As weigh-ins for a tournament or a meet approach, many of my teammates brag about not having eaten for 24 hours or longer, highlighting their ability to starve their bodies and shed unhealthy amounts of weight in a short time...I never once interacted with a sports dietician or someone specifically trained to support athletes with disordered eating.

Like many health teachers who teach prescribed or outdated curriculum, "athletic trainer[s] and coaches have a base level understanding of nutrition and disordered eating."[315]

Another piece of advice Kayla Stansberry mentioned in our conversation is to not comment on student athletes' bodies at all, and to focus instead on skill building in a particular sport. "I notice you got faster" is a lot different than "you ran faster in this race because you lost weight" (again, the lighter = faster implication of track and cross country is right there). Focusing on what athletes do, how they improve or change their skill level over time, takes the focus off the body by decoupling the correlation between ability, athleticism, and size.

If you are coaching a sport, make it about building strength and building connection instead of changing their body. Coaches should have training and education about how to talk about (or not talk about) food and bodies. Saying things like "make sure your thighs don't get too big," is advice that will ring in athletes' minds for life.

Eating Disorders and Disordered Eating: The Difference

Eating disorders are specific sets of criteria and behavior that yield a medical diagnosis. They create long-term and short-term health risks, especially for kids who are not finished growing yet, as we saw with the female athlete triad earlier in this chapter. Disordered eating, on the other hand, is a subclinical pattern of behaviors related to food and body image, which may include eliminating entire food groups or refusal to eat certain foods because they are perceived to make someone gain weight, or skipping social events where food is a focus, or spending a seemingly obsessive amount of time planning meals.[317]

The language of disordered eating shows up in coaching and guidance around nutrition, even if it's well intended. "Lighter equals faster" often came about in the form of food policing, body policing, in the warmups where coaches shouted "engage your core!" or workouts after practice formally ended. For athletes who are restricting and bingeing to manipulate weight, many use the term "cheat meal" to refer to going off script from a restrictive meal plan or eating food that is low in "desirable" macronutrients. In fact, people who are likely to associate certain foods with "guilt" end up gaining weight over time.[318] Kayla Stansberry spoke with me about how athletic advisors, coaches, and staff can make changes in these areas: "If we're villainizing sugars and fats, we already have that attachment to those foods and what they mean about larger bodied people," she said.

> **Quick Tip**
>
> *Instead of diet, referring to meals as a "meal plan" may take the diet culture out of food.*

When we put morality onto food, children cannot comprehend that aggressive of a duality – when we say kids shouldn't have sugar, they are internalizing messages of good and bad when it comes to food. It's not an individual issue, it's a systemic issue. The way we talk about food is normalized, so everyone does it. Having a different, gentler understanding of nutrition all around.

Who Run the World? Girl (Scouts)

Though not affiliated in any official or extracurricular capacity with schools, a common extracurricular activity that kids are joining is Scouts. Girl Scouts USA boasts a membership of 2.5 million, including more than 1.7 million scouts and 750,000 adults.[319] Most of what people know about Girl Scouts is that they do community service, empower, and encourage girls and women everywhere, and that, of course, they sell cookies.

Almost inevitably, diet culture shows up in Girl Scout cookie sales. Writers craft entire think pieces about Girl Scout cookies, obesity, dieting, and "moderation" around cookie season. Jokes like "will these Thin Mints make me thin?" and comments like "I can't have those in the house, I'll eat the whole box in one day!" when someone leaves a sign up sheet in the break room, just feels like part of the Girl Scout cookie enjoying experience. [320] Admittedly, when cookie season came around this year, I bought a lot of boxes, specifically to support LGBTQIA+ scouts in queer-unfriendly places like Ohio, in pursuing trips and community service projects. After that, my local troop was selling boxes outside of our local supermarket, and instead of purchasing more, I dropped money in the jar to donate. Moderation around Girl Scout cookies is entirely possible, and acting like they are this forbidden food – especially when variations of them are available year round in the Cookie aisle – does not do anyone any good, especially when folks verbalize that diet talk aloud for all colleagues to hear.

In my research about Girl Scouts, I could not find any similar critique about Boy Scouts popcorn sales – no one is worried about what their $25 canisters of popcorn will do to your waistline. In recent years, there have even been false rumors circulated by right-wing anti-choice groups that Girl Scout cookie sales fund abortion.[321] This rumor started in 2004, when the leader of an anti-abortion group in Waco, Texas went on Christian radio to protest a "cozy relationship" between Girl Scouts USA and Planned Parenthood. The rumor began when the Bluebonnet Council, a group that included area scout troops, had its name and logo on brochures distributed at a Planned Parenthood sex education program for young people. Since then, the falsehood that Girl Scouts and Planned Parenthood are financially connected has circulated, with anti-abortion activists vowing to boycott the cookie sales each year.[321]

Girl Scouts USA has repeatedly proven through their tax forms that they are not affiliated in any way with Planned Parenthood, financially or otherwise.

> From 5-year-old Daisies to 16-year-old Senior Scouts, girls are often forced to bear the brunt of angry tirades from adults who want to lecture them about healthy eating, moan about price hikes, or rant about the group's rumored (and false) link to Planned Parenthood,

said Lela Moore for an article in *Business Insider*.[321] Both of these points, when taken together, illustrate the barrage of criticism often only afforded to girls and women. Girl Scouts are to blame for everything from our cookie indulgences to reproductive healthcare. It's misogyny, plain, and simple. "Given that over 200 million boxes of cookies are sold each year, that's a lot of girls fending off a lot of snarky remarks about bathing suit season or earning the confection through extra workouts or starvation," said Dr. Katie Hurley in a 2023 article for *CNN*.[322]

The same girls who are learning entrepreneurial skills from Girl Scout cookie sales are also subject constantly to diet culture, and the expectation to start worrying about fat, calories, and weight from an early age. Oona Hanson, who we've heard from a lot throughout this book, says about it in an essay:

> Because these kinds of remarks are repeated and concentrated into a short period of time, they can really do a number on a child's perceptions of food and bodies. And the comments don't have to be menacing or self-righteous to cause harm. Even the seemingly innocuous self-deprecating humor can worm its way into a child's sense of how they should relate to their own body.[320]

One example of this happening is troop mom Morgan Shelly, from Shaker Heights, Ohio, who, in 2016 ran a supermarket cookie booth with her troop of fourth- and fifth-grade scouts. She said that during their sales shift, one woman "looked at the girls and just responded, 'Cookies make you fat.' And walked away."[321] Moms like Jamie Davis Smith, who wrote about her experience for Yahoo!, said that Girl Scouts helped her stop talking about weight to and around her kids, especially in a negative way. Her daughter came home and reported that "around 30" people told her daughter at the cookie booth that they "shouldn't buy the cookies because they were trying to lose weight."[323]

Comments like this cause troop leaders to have to work hard to undo the harm. One comment may last a few seconds, and cookie sales happen once a year – but diet culture's hurt is permanent and lasting. When things like this happen, troop leaders may take up meeting time to educate girls about diet culture and anti-fat bias; and, since many adults are still living and breathing in the same anti-fatness they learned as children, it can be a learning experience for everyone to take on together. The Girl Scouts organization even has a badge for that; the "Free to be Me" module teaches self-esteem and body positivity. However, according to Hanson, they also have some nutrition education that plays on problematic language about weight, so she recommends proceeding with caution in those areas.[320]

No Fortunate Sons

According to its own promotional materials, the Junior Reserve Officer Training Corps (JROTC) is "an exciting program offered to high school students that teaches character education, student achievement, health and wellness, leadership and diversity." In both English and Spanish, they explain "how it works," with an emphasis on citizenship and patriotism.[324]

The Department of Defense touts the Army JROTC program as, in their own words, being "one of the few programs available in the school schedule that has such a profound impact on motivating students to excel."[324] JROTC also prepares students for "postsecondary options including college or the workforce. Through cadet-run programs and team competitions, students learn invaluable professional skills like leadership, teamwork, time-management, self-discipline and communication." The program emphasizes these qualities, including physical fitness to prospective cadet recruits.

None of these values or characteristics is a bad thing on their own, but when examining the methods used to recruit cadets into JROTC programs and into the military in general, there are practices that are problematic at best and sinister at worst. The language of "self-discipline" shows up a lot, and often, those who are the most recruited into these programs are students of color. When coupled with who is most targeted for recruitment (youth of color from poor households)[325], it suggests that these students lack self-discipline, academic and interpersonal skills, and that the DOD is the institution that can teach them these values. The same kind of "discipline" rhetoric is often pushed onto fat bodies, and for the same reasons. For thousands of students across America, it was reported in a New York Times investigation, students have been forced to join the program, which is not forbidden, though discouraged, by the military itself. This led to President Biden having to sign a law banning forced enrollment in 2024.[326] The investigation into forced recruitment came on the heels of another investigation into sexual abuse and misconduct by JROTC training instructors, who usually serve as employees of the school districts where they work. Since 2017, allegations against 58 individual JROTC instructors across branches – 26 Army JROTC (all but one substantiated), 16 Marine Corps JROTC (all substantiated), 11 Navy JROTC (all but one substantiated) and seven Air Force JROTC (all substantiated) – were corroborated by law enforcement or school officials. Questioning and moderating these programs in schools is, then, not only a matter of keeping kids safe from predatory messages about diet culture, fitness, nationalism, and militarization, but safe violence and abuse as well.[327]

Another means of ensuring "discipline" in these students is to turn them into "warriors." Students get to carry titles like "battalion commander" and participate in local parades and "elegant" military balls.[324] If we think back to Dr. Oz's comments about fitness being the ultimate act of patriotism, it makes sense that they'd use fat as a scapegoat for why military recruitment numbers are dwindling. And JROTC becomes ever more important to changing that, in the eyes of the DoD, considering that "just over a third of young adults ages 17–24 are too heavy to serve in the military." [328] To boost recruitment efforts, the military "granted enlistment waivers for recruits with a body composition of up to 2% body fat over the accession standard if recruits could pass a physical endurance, motivation and strength assessment." Even in our armed forces, they recognized that weight was not a determination of strength, stamina, and endurance – but not necessarily because they believed in fat people's ability – because they needed numbers. Reports by the military's own health system indicate that from 2017 to 2021, the incidence of eating disorders increased among servicemembers by 79 percent. [328]

According to Steve Beynon,

> JROTC is a program funded by the Pentagon designed to teach basic civics and leadership skills – all while subtly pitching military service to those students through trips to military bases, doing military-style physical challenges like obstacle courses, and having them occasionally wear uniforms. JROTC units are commonplace in parades and other military ceremonies to give those students a taste of the culture. [326]

Though there is no requirement to enlist or even to continue on to ROTC college programs, roughly 20–25 percent of JROTC/ROTC cadets enlist and serve the military in some capacity. [326] Today, there are just over 1,700 Army JROTC programs in the United States, with approximately 275,000 cadets. About 280 schools are on a "wait list" to establish their own programs, costing the Army only about $800 per cadet each year out of approximately a $200 million budget. [326] These programs share many of their costs with the school districts themselves, who enter into an agreement through annual budgets for the program. Many students from poor families, especially students of color, join because doing so makes access to college and healthcare less burdensome, because ROTC programs that recruit and train officers for enlistment into the armed services offer to pay for their tuition, textbooks, and other costs. In many cases, it serves as a pipeline to financial stability that many without generational wealth would otherwise not be able to access, but in turn, it serves as a pipeline to the military-industrial complex. In a 2017 RAND study, they found that 55 percent of the schools in America with a JROTC program were Title I eligible, meaning they had a high number or a majority of students living in poverty.[329] At schools with JROTC programs, 56.6 percent of students on average are eligible for free and reduced lunch based on family income. At public high schools without JROTC programs, an average of 46.9 percent of students are eligible for free or reduced-price lunch.[329]

And, according to their own reports, young people don't want to join the military regardless of their fitness level or eligibility. A 2020 poll found that only 11 percent of respondents ages 16–24 said they were "likely" to serve in the military in the next few years.[330] Whether because they are fat, unmotivated, or just plain not buying what the military is selling them, this generation of students is less interested in signing up to become even a small part of the war machine.

After-school programming and extracurriculars like scouts, clubs, sports, and theater can be a powerful place for kids to find belonging and see school as a net positive experience. Making sure those spaces are also minimizing the ways that they internalize weight stigma can ensure that students have more positive experiences in school than negative ones.

RUN IT BACK – Reflecting on Your Practice

◆ *How does anti-fatness look differently in extracurricular spaces than in academic ones? How does it look the same?*
◆ *Do we have extracurricular activities at my school that emphasize joy and not just competition?*

♦ *How can my school support its extracurricular programs and facilitators in eliminating and calling in anti-fat bias, and other oppressions, with fidelity?*

♦ *Does our school district have explicit policies safeguarding against language or practices that encourage disordered eating or negative body image beyond the classroom?*

♦ *How are the ways that anti-fat bias shows up gendered, abled, or racialized in these spaces? How can we, as a school or district, do our "table work" around these issues?*

♦ *Do we need to consider or reconsider our relationship with organizations, contractors, or people who bring diet talk, negative body image or fatphobia into our space?*

III

The Remix

The chapters in Part III of this book will focus on the teacher-facing parts of how fatphobia happens at school, and how teachers and building leaders can support the adults in dismantling anti-fatness so that the kids will be alright.

DOI: 10.4324/9781003534143-10

8

Workin' 7-3

Anti-Fat Bias and the Teacher Day

Presently, there are no federal U.S. laws that protect people from weight-based discrimination, including in the workplace. Only a handful of cities and states have such legislation or policy on the books.[331] In an age where the media, politicians, and their followers demonize diversity, equity and inclusion work on a regular basis, the push to make workspaces more inclusive for anyone, let alone for fat people, is tenuous at best. Michigan was the first state to ban weight-based discrimination, and in 2019, Washington state followed suit. In New York City, Mayor Eric Adams signed a law in 2023 to ban weight- and height-based discrimination.[298]

Like Beverly Daniel Tatum, the author of *Why Are All the Black Kids Sitting Together In the Cafeteria?*, says about white supremacy, fatphobia is in the air we breathe.[297] Anti-fat bias has barraged all of us for our entire lives. And while it is far from the "last acceptable form of oppression," it remains one of the toughest, in my opinion, to unlearn, because it happens inside and around racism, ableism, sexism, classism, and all other oppressions that exist to create the systems we live and teach in. So it makes sense that for teachers, it would show up at work. Studies have shown

DOI: 10.4324/9781003534143-11

that fat women are three times more likely than men to report discrimination in the hiring process, especially when a position involves building personal relationships, being visible to the public, or requiring physical demands. In education, many teachers are fat; and especially at the early childhood level,[332] probably for a few reasons. One, because fat women are often seen as caretakers due to their social invisibility, placing others' needs before their own. Two, because society undervalues caretaking, and education in general, but especially preschool settings which are often considered "childcare," despite the many motor skills, social and play skills, and early literacy skills taught by daycare and preschool professionals. Three, because the way that our society devalues the voices and inherent worth of children, despite incessantly claiming that they are our "future." Often, fat teachers, too, are at the bottom of a social hierarchy. Fat people, generally, are not given jobs that include fostering relationships or being publicly visible. When we apply this to a school, fat people are less visible in administrative roles, but make up much of the teaching profession. We are "good enough" to teach and have authority over children, but not "good enough" to make school policy decisions, lead, or foster school culture from a position of influence like the principal's office or superintendency. And when we do, the double trouble of being catapulted from invisibility to hypervisibility – that is, every decision we make that someone disagrees with, or every misstep or misspeak – is doubly judged for its content on top of who we are as people while making those decisions. This is especially true of fat women of color in leadership roles.

American society holds its teachers to an impossible standard, especially those in marginalized positions. Queer teachers are regularly subject to double standards at work for how much they share their personal lives with students. Though it wasn't always the case, the same is not true of many or most straight educators, who have family photos visible in their classrooms and go out on maternity or paternity leave. In a similar way, society perceives fat teachers as "setting a bad example for kids," especially if they are fat and in positions where they teach health or physical education.

One study in 2020 published in *Preventive Medicine Reports* surveyed teachers from a mid-Atlantic state, asking teachers to respond to questions like "I let my students drink water in class," "I eat healthy meals or snacks in front of my students during the school day," and "I care about making my school a healthier place."[333] The study was sponsored by the USDA and the American Heart Association, among other organizations, and the findings suggest that teachers' diet quality is poor, largely, it says, due to purchasing snacks and sugary drinks from vending machines throughout the school day. The researchers concluded in the results that "teachers had fairly unhealthy personal dietary habits, and those with the least healthy diets were more likely to engage in classroom practices that could adversely impact their students' dietary patterns." The study neglects to mention things that are entirely out of teacher's control, such as their own genetics, and the social determinants of health in both their own lives and the lives of their students.[333]

I've actually had acquaintances lament to me about their kid's "overweight" gym teacher, saying things like "What could they possibly teach my kid about health if they're so fat?" They also said that their child, whom they encouraged to be fatphobic, reported that the teacher "ate McDonald's every day." I did not know this teacher, so I cannot confirm or deny this recollection; but what I can report is that the way it was said leaned more toward it being a trope weaponized to express dislike for the teacher rather than having a basis in observable fact. Fatness is often a proxy for our disdain, because it's easier to demean or dehumanize someone if they somehow "deserve" it due to their perceived lack of ability, their weight, their size, their supposed laziness, or all the above.

Before criticizing teachers for their food choices, it's important to note that the average American school teacher makes nearly a thousand decisions in a single school day.[334] Sometimes, those decisions involve using the small window of time you have between periods to make copies or use the bathroom. Teachers are, for the most part, a mix of sedentary and mobile throughout their day. Especially elementary school teachers, who often have to shuttle students back and forth from recess, specials, and other activities, often build movement into their day somewhat intrinsically. We do not always have schedules that enable us to prioritize self-care or basic needs. The expectation to keep going after contractual hours to complete grades, enter progress report comments, and correspond with parents, remains a part of the culture of education. If you're a teacher reading this, you know what working through lunch to get grading done so you can spend time with your family, and thus, foregoing a fully balanced meal to do so, feels like. You know the teacher's guilt of making sure students have enough feedback to improve on their next essay. All these things are a function of misogyny – the expectation that teachers, who work in a profession dominated by women, are on the go and committed to their work of assessing, teaching, caring for, and shaping the lives of other peoples' children. Self-care falls by the wayside all too often – and it is not our personal responsibility to change the system that makes this true and possible. These changes have to come from systems, from administrators, and from school culture.

Educators are expected to be "on" all the time. Many consider us to be performers, actors, facilitators – all roles that require active engagement and openness in front of a collective audience. But does it all have to happen while standing?

In her essay "On Being a Fat Preschool Teacher," Haven Mitchell-Rose asserts that

> to be a teacher is to be hyper-visible. You are on display all day in front of a group of children who spend a lot of time looking at you. As one of the few adults they consistently interact with, you are a role model for these kids.

In describing her experience, Mitchell-Rose highlights the multifacetedness of teaching while fat: being subject to visibility of appearance, but invisibility of voice, and often. Being expected to be a role model, but seen as a "bad influence" on kids just for existing. As one-dimensional as representation on its own may be and feel, it can have a healing effect for so many different reasons in the classroom. Haven says,

I remind myself that I have the power to be for my students what I needed so badly as a kid: a role model for radical body acceptance, and in my best moments, for fat joy and pride…in having me as their teacher during these early formative years, my students are seeing a competent fat person in action, living a successful and fulfilling life, and hopefully forming an association that extends beyond me and to the other fat folks they encounter.[335]

There are many reasons to move around a classroom space while teaching; checking for understanding, engaging in feedback and conferencing, and helping students remain on task or engaged in the day's lesson. Especially for students who need more scaffolds for attention and focus, a sort of "body double" circulating the room is helpful and can remind them to give all their attention to what they're learning. Standing, walking, and moving have become synonymous with active, "good" teaching, whereas teachers who sit are perceived as less active.

The same can be said of our students, in the converse: the "ideal" learner is seated, attentive, participating, and helping us move the lesson along; they don't disrupt or distract others with their words or their movements. While proximity to the teacher is helpful, I have often found that students see it as a mechanism for monitoring their behavior in ways that demand compliance, and don't necessarily always facilitate focus and learning; instead, it creates a climate where the pressure to complete tasks under the watchful eye of the educator, not necessarily learning, is at the forefront of the teacher's presence in the room. On the other side of the coin, expecting students to remain seated, which they do for approximately 70 percent of their school day, may not be conducive to cognitive input and retention. The perception that students must sit while learning and that teachers must be standing while teaching boils down to power dynamics: teacher as expert and authority, student as subject. And classroom "management" built on control and power struggles, rather than collaborative relationships, makes room for assumptions about teachers who remain seated while teaching to be viewed as less effective.[336]

My friend and fellow educator Alex Shevrin Venet told me,

> In the context of a classroom, teachers *are* required to supervise our classes, and sometimes this does involve being positioned so we can see everyone. But there isn't a binary of choices between "walking around and standing constantly" and "unable to see and supervise my students." I've used tall chairs to get a good vantage point of the room, rotated students through groups with me while I remained in one spot, and used mobility tools such as a rollator if I did need to circulate a room.

According to an article from the British Council,

> Whilst sitting down in front of students at the beginning of a class can create a welcoming, cozy atmosphere, if we are not careful, remaining seated throughout the class can give students the impression of a lack of interest and motivation on our part.[337]

These assumptions about teachers who sit while teaching land most insidiously on teachers in larger bodies and teachers with invisible disabilities: the assumption is that we are lazy, less motivated, less "in control" of a classroom, and less good at our jobs.

To this notion, Alex adds,

> Standing up isn't morally superior to sitting down – that's an ableist idea. Instead, let's focus on the actual goals: building relationships, supervising the class safely, conferencing with students about their work, or whatever it may be – and use all the tools available to us to best match our bodies' needs to those tasks.

Mobility looks different for everyone, and isn't indicative of a person's willingness to engage with others or their ability to help students learn.

Also as of 2024, more and more teachers are impacted by long-COVID and continue to be exposed to the virus in schools. "It's safe to assume," says Texas ELA teacher Chanea Bond, "that some teachers will become chronically ill. Expecting those teachers to stand is ableism that is not conducive to a teaching environment." As policy and media sentiment shift to tell us that the pandemic days are over, for many of us, they are not.

Just like there is no universal experience of living in a larger body, there is no universal experience of ability. Plenty of fat bodies can move and move agilely; they're just larger while they move. Yet, we treat people in larger bodies as if the fact of their size is in and of itself a disability, and use that to question their competence, physical capacity, and more. This is both fatphobia and ableism at work. Negative attitudes toward fat bodies are ever-present in the media that we all consume, and are in the curriculum and institutional layout of our schools. It is possible to teach, and teach well, sitting down.

One of the reasons I suggest that anti-fat bias is among the toughest social biases to unlearn (though not the last "acceptable" one by any stretch, especially in a world full of racism, ableism, and other forms of discrimination) is that, related to intersectionality, is this simple fact: 80 percent of the people who make up the teaching profession today are white, and a majority of those who teach are also women. While women are, in varying and different degrees, subject to misogyny, beauty standards, and gender-based discrimination, white women have benefited from the parts of white supremacy that still remain intact today. Linked here is the fact that since the time of the transatlantic slave trade, when white enslavers assigned characteristics that distinguished the slaves they bought and sold as inferior – introducing colorism, and then supposing that Black bodies were fatter and more sexualized because they lacked discipline and control.[16, 229] Thus, even in a teaching profession marked by the immense and disproportionate labor of women in general, white women are overrepresented in education as a whole.

What it looks like now is that those who are the most marginalized are "becoming" fat at higher rates. When examining the causation and correlation of an increase in fatness with a decrease in socioeconomic status (meaning the poorest Americans are living in increasingly larger bodies), we must note that "scientists" used the same rhetoric to vilify and demean Black bodies a century ago.[338] This fallacy assumes poor people are "uneducated" about nutrition and health, and those who make these assumptions overlook factors such as genetics, built environment. In the case of teachers who live in fat bodies, the limited prep time, the expectation to work through lunch or after school and the lack of work-life balance that causes many to burn out quickly may be worth studying. In an article for *Rethinking Schools*, teacher Reuben Abrahams Brosbe says:

> Like so many other forms of oppression prevalent in the United States, fatphobia imparts shame and failure on us by placing the burden for wellness on us as individuals rather than the systems we live under. This is a recurring tool of social control under racial capitalism. Diet culture would have us believe that the key to health is in our personal choices about what we eat, how much we eat, and whether we move our bodies enough in certain ways.[339]

As the number of fat people in America has increased, so has anti-fat bias. Reports indicate that more than 40 percent of adults in the United States have experienced weight-related stigma at some point in their lives. At work, this can take the form of microaggressions.[239]

Being Quiet Is Free

If you've heard someone say "You're eating a salad – that's way better than what I have today," or "I'm not going to eat any of those cookies left out from the party – I'm trying to *be good*," you may at least begin to see what I mean. In spaces where women are often expected to work more and still make less, grade and plan past contract hours, and compete in a teacher shortage for employment and tenure, sexism and the transmutation of mom guilt to teacher guilt run rampant, leaving little time for self-care, meals, and bathroom breaks. As we've explored in previous chapters, thin supremacy is a close relative of white supremacy. And when you put all of that together, you get attempts at oppressive solidarity – a group of people trying to relate to each other by hating their bodies. It's a form of social bonding that is not exclusive to, but common among, women, and since that's who most of who's in the teaching profession, it is in the air that we breathe in faculty rooms, team meetings, and staff celebrations. In her article for LinkedIn, recruiting specialist Michelle Duffie states, "If a 'compliment' projects societal insecurities onto someone else, is it really a compliment?"[340] This kind of social bonding creates a culture that is implicitly and explicitly hostile to fat bodies, and, by extension, disabled and racialized bodies as well, because it considers and codifies what (and who) is superior, what/who is "good," and puts anything else into the binary category of "bad/other."

When phrases like "I'm being good" or the urge to compare lunches are put into the air, what's actually being said, albeit quietly, is that there's judgment and shame for anyone who *does* eat the leftover cookies or bring in a plate of pasta. What's felt, no matter how unintentionally, is a wide gap of moral fortitude between the person being "good" and anyone who dares to bring in cake. Of course, it may remain in the environments we teach and live in because it feels futile to fight it and gargantuan to unlearn. In an article for *Security Management Magazine*, Anna Burns says, "Because it's so accepted and ingrained in our culture, anti-fat bias is the norm, and in my experience, no time, place or space is immune from it entirely."[239]

Simply put: being quiet is free. We don't have to verbalize our discontent with our bodies just because, and expect everyone to join in. We can keep our thoughts about the cake to ourselves, or, at worst, if we feel like we can't help but have an unplanned slice, walk out and eat what we brought to work somewhere else. Faculty spaces are spaces for building community, socializing, venting, copying (the Xerox kind, not the mimicking diet culture talking points kind), and prepping and planning. Stray diet comments, food policing, and body shame can make these sacred teacher spaces less safe and inclusive for everyone in them, including those who are still stuck in diet land. In her podcast *Burnt Toast*, Virginia Sole-Smith articulates a point worth considering:

> If the core of fat liberation is body autonomy, then we have to keep making space for everybody gets to make their own choices for their bodies, but I do think we have a responsibility to each other in how we talk about those choices.[341]

There is plenty of research that points to the pervasiveness of negative body talk and its impact on mental health. A 2011 study found that those who overheard negative body talk were more likely to participate in it, especially if nobody challenged them either privately or publicly.[342] A 2003 study in the International Journal of Eating Disorders found that as little as three to five minutes of negative body discussion can impact a person's body image, or even, in the case of those with eating disorders, their recovery.[342] This is especially important to consider when we are around students who are still developing their body image and identity, but it can certainly have a negative impact on the adults around us, too. A "culture of consent" around everything, including body talk in the workplace, can help to create more inclusive spaces that prioritize the well-being of adults, whose mental and physical health is often sidelined at school.

If it feels like you are in a position to educate others in the moment, refer them to the ASDAH definition of health or resources on the social determinants of health. ASDAH refers to health as

> a holistic definition that cannot be characterized simply as the absence of a physical or mental illness, limitation, or disease. Rather, health exists on a continuum that varies with time and circumstances for each individual. Health should not be conceived as a resource or capacity available to all, regardless of condition or ability level, and not as an outcome or objective of living. Pursuing health is

neither a moral imperative nor an individual obligation, and health status should never be used to judge, oppress, or determine the value of an individual.[343]

In general, it's not good workplace practice to talk about anyone's bodies, whether you believe you're paying them a compliment or not. Impact far outweighs intention. Just like in conversations about racism or other types of oppression, our desire to distance ourselves from having implicit bias does not go away when we're engaging in body talk. The backhanded "You're not fat, you're beautiful," exists on the same plane as trying to backflip your way out of believing and reinforcing racialized stereotypes because you have close friends or colleagues of color. Our privilege does not change in proximity to people who have less of it, and neither does the necessity that we unlearn, unpack, and listen.

And if someone is trying to redirect negative body talk or to tell you that casual comment was fatphobic, believe them. It is often a reflex to say "I didn't mean it like that," but as we tell students all the time – words have meaning, and we are responsible for our actions. This book aims to prioritize anti-fat bias in the context of intrapersonal, interpersonal, and institutional[343] bias and harm because it *is* harmful. And while all bodies deserve and need to be free from shame at work and at school, some bodies are subject to more fear, hate, shame, and violence than others.

That's why, when someone tells you about anti-fat bias happening to them, "Skinny shaming matters too," isn't an appropriate response. Thin bodies are, whether they feel it or not, given the societal standard of more value, more worth, and, in the case of work, more money. Individualized aggressions toward thin people are equally inappropriate, but they do not reach the same level of institutional, systemically exclusive bias that becomes policy against fat bodies. In a 2020 essay, Aubrey Gordon stated.

Those individual, interpersonal instances are different than being denied the ability to meet even your most basic needs. Being told to "eat something" is jarring and unkind, the kind of unbidden comment that can stay with you for months, days or even years. It is a different problem than a court ruling that it's not illegal to fire someone for gaining weight…It is different than requiring job applicants to meet or fall below a certain BMI.[344]

In conversations where people attempt to one-up each other's negative lived experiences or bond over body shame, thin people may express very real, very upsetting instances of body shaming. They may also believe that, in their heart, they are being kind when they tell a fat colleague that they "look great," followed by "Did you lose weight?" or tell a fat colleague who refers to themselves as fat that they're "not fat, they're beautiful." These kinds of comments come from the false belief that it's better, and worth celebrating, and more attractive, to be smaller. And when we ask a skinny person "what's your secret!?" the "secret" may very well be an eating disorder, an underlying illness, invisible disability, or chemotherapy side effects.

In her interview for the *Food Psych* podcast with Christy Harrison, Sofie Hagen said aptly:

> We've spent a lot of energy saying no, I'm not privileged and I'm not racist and I'm not I'm not I'm not, and I think the only way we can really actually get through this is by going we have all learned these things and we all encompass them in some way…and we can't fix that unless we acknowledge that we all have it [implicit bias].[343]

In their book *Thinfluence: The Powerful and Surprising Effect Friends, Family, Work and Environment have on Weight*, Doctors Walter Willett and Malissa Wood suggest that "food pushers" and external influences have an inordinate amount of influence on our ability to stay thin. "Sometimes," they say, "this happens without our even knowing it, especially since while we are at work, the task at hand often seems more important than paying attention to actions that might be affecting our weight."[345]

The researchers, both employed at Harvard Medical School, toe the line of diet culture and personal responsibility in their book.

> A song or office celebration on a birthday can go a long way in terms of making someone feel appreciated. A regularly scheduled office night out or working lunch is great for team morale. But the way these occasions are celebrated or enjoyed is often the problem…a slice of birthday cake is about three hundred calories, give or take. So if you have twenty employees where you work, all of whom have birthdays, that's six thousand extra calories per year in birthday cake alone.[345]

They're offering, they suggest, not a lesson in calorie counting, but an illustration of "how pressure to be part of the team can often mean pressure to fit in and indulge." Their solutions range from "encouraging healthy competition," buying a FitBit, getting a treadmill desk (which retails at about $800–$2500) or a pedal exerciser ($40), and "finding a "Thinfluencer" in your workplace – someone who makes the "right choices involving diet, exercise, and attitude." The authors encourage readers who are stuck in a "nutritionally hostile" work environment to "form a small group to try and help each other make the right choices."[345] But what are the right choices, exactly? Those differ, nutritionally, socially, and culturally, for everyone.

What the authors are suggesting is a form of *concern trolling* – and may end up making the workplace more hostile than if you just packed your lunch or minded your business. Concern trolling is "when someone feigns support for a cause or group while subtly undermining it through fabricated concerns or criticisms."[346] Under the guise of "caring" about employees' health, initiatives that center on weight loss are subtly (or sometimes not so subtly) telling employees that they "should" lose weight. This kind of attitude can create environments where the space subjects fat people, or even those with perceived proximity to fatness, to their food choices, normalizes environments of unsolicited health and weight loss advice that feel pointed, and makes work a less effective, less safe place for all. That "healthy competition" to get more steps in may not be accessible to your colleagues who use mobility devices, and thus ends up being exclusionary. I'd argue that concern trolling is a form of workplace harassment; it creates environments openly hostile to fat people, under the banner of healthism. Aubrey Gordon states

> Programs that offer financial or health care incentives for meeting biometric targets tend to systematically disadvantage people who are already disabled or chronically ill. For example, those with advanced diabetes may not be able to meet a blood glucose target designed for nondiabetic people.[347]

What these workplace wellness initiatives fail to account for are the social determinants of health, which account for up to 70 percent of a person's modifiable health outcomes.[343] What this means is that individual behaviors, like diet and exercise, account for only about 30 percent of our ability to control our weight. So, putting the onus on employees to "control their weight" and therefore control costs is not only statistically destined for failure, but it's also bad policy that can lower work morale overall. They assume everyone starts in the same place, but fail to take into account access to things like education, fresh food, built environments, and physical and interpersonal safety.

Instead of building an environment of exclusion in the name of fitness, we can build a culture of consent around body talk and opt for inclusion and belonging. The profession at large asks teachers to sacrifice so much for their students, including their well-being; the least we can do is care for each other's mental health by not including body talk in our daily interactions with one another. In another article for SELF, Aubrey Gordon discusses healthism, which we defined in Chapter 1 and discussed in Chapter 3. She says that concern trolling like the kind mentioned in *Thinfluence,* contains "clear and implicit judgment: you're doing it wrong. You have failed. I have been monitoring your health. I know your body better than you," under a guise of caring concern.[348]

Healthism isn't just a problem for fat people – it's a tool used to further anti-fat bias, yes, but also ableism, transphobia, misogyny, racism and more. Healthism shows up when we joke about getting diabetes from a single dessert, or refer to a rich meal as a "heart attack on a plate" – implying that those health conditions are caused by failures of a perceived personal responsibility to be healthy, not by structural forces that disproportionately harm the health of people living on the down side of power.[348]

While healthism is a learned behavior, Gordon says, "it's one that also often gives us a sense of mastery, control over our own bodies, and sometimes, a sense of superiority over those whose health we're so ready to judge."[348] It creates less connection, less collaboration, and ultimately, less productivity at our jobs when we make other people small by suggesting that they become smaller, for no other reason than that's what we believe they *should* be doing.

> **Quick Tip**
>
> *Some ways to interrupt diet talk can include changing the subject, setting firm boundaries ("I don't want to engage in that kind of talk about food or bodies here," or (with permission) offering resources like this book to change and reframe thinking around diet, weight, and body image.*

A Hard Day's Fight

Alongside teachers generally being paid less than other professions and largely undervalued before and after the COVID-19 pandemic, it's true that fat people make less money than their thin counterparts. Companies are also less likely to hire fat people, specifically women, in public-facing positions such as in education, administrative, or superintendent roles. In general, some research has even showed that even just slightly fatter people make up to $9,000 less annually than their thin colleagues.[347] According to Matt Gonzalez in an article for the Society for Human Resources Management, the "weight penalty," like the gender pay gap, is difficult to track down, because salary goes down as weight goes up; meaning that in some cases, schools may not expect or encourage a teacher in a larger body to negotiate their salary, and thus start in lower places than their thin colleagues despite the same or more experience.[331] When it comes to pay, the biggest disparity in the "weight penalty" gap hurts fat women at work. "Just a ten percent increase in body mass can result in a six percent reduction in salary for women, according to research cited by NPR."[239] Research done by SRHM showed that employees in larger bodies, in general, are more likely to be perceived as lazy, unmotivated, and unprofessional, while "average" weight employees are perceived as high performing, hard working and motivated.[239] These findings are similar to the perceptions that teachers have of students in larger bodies about their intelligence, student skills, and work ethic that we discussed in the early chapters of this book.

Eleven percent of HR professionals have reported that an applicant's weight has played a role in decisions their organizations (including schools) have made during the job application process. In another study, 45 percent of employers indicated that they were "less inclined" to hire candidates who are fat.[338] And as of right now, there is not much that prospective or current employees can do about it in court. Rebecca Puhl, whose work we've seen in previous chapters, was quoted in an article saying,

> Weight discrimination can be present in different ways in the workplace, including unfair hiring practices, such as refusing to hire qualified job applicants because of their body size; fewer promotions; stigma or stereotypes from coworkers and supervisors; and wrongful job termination.[239]

She also noted that "such discrimination can also be manifested in more subtle, difficult-to-prove ways at work, such as assigning office chairs that cannot accommodate employees with larger bodies or failing to provide accessible bathroom stalls."[239]

But it can also be even more subtle than that. Chairs with arms in the faculty lounge can create uncomfortable and even altogether inaccessible spaces for meetings, teaching, or prep. Ordering furniture without arms, chairs, and couches that sit higher off the ground, and sitting equipment with higher weight capacities can help to ensure that no one is humiliated for trying to do the basic tasks of their job.

Another subtle way it shows up is in school swag orders. Those PTA-sponsored school stores, that sometimes only go up to a 2X, are not inclusive of everyone. Allowing people to decide for themselves what size they wear, and asking for size orders instead of bulk ordering a set amount of each size in advance, is a way to ensure that everyone is included – especially if staff wear apparel on designated days of the week or for special events. Unisex clothing is also a good way to ensure that more inclusive sizing is used, because gendered clothing is cut differently and may not fit.[340] If your school store only carries up to a certain size, advocate that they extend the sizing, even if it means spending a little extra – it's worth the price of inclusion.

> **Quick Tip**
>
> *Ask your Board of Education, building administration, and union what the policies are against weight discrimination. If your school, union, or district doesn't have those yet, offer to help write one or start the conversation.*

How Hard Should We Be Working on Our Fitness?

A 2013 report found that 16 percent of workplaces require wellness programs.[349] But when employers connect those programs explicitly to weight loss initiatives (as 67 percent of company wellness programs are), they can produce effects that have nothing to do with health. Union-sponsored health insurance, in my case, has an option to pay for my gym membership, which can be a great way to make exercise and movement affordable for so many. I'm lucky enough that that doesn't come with constant emails about wellness and weight loss, as some insurance and employee assistance programs do.

Some schools, however, have hosted and promoted their own "Biggest Loser" competitions among staff, encouraging several weeks of sustained weight loss including weigh-ins, with the results publicly posted. For example, Altoona Area

High School hosted one in 2024, in which staff competed to lose weight for nine weeks in 18 teams of four and reported their weights in the nurse's office.[350] Other schools that created similar competitions include Dearborn Schools. In their 2016 version of the competition, teachers paid an entry fee, paid per weigh-in, and winners received a $200 gift card (first place) $100 gift card (second place), or a $50 gift card (third place) for losing the most body weight.[351] Using the Biggest Loser event as a model, the University of Oklahoma created student math worksheet materials with participant faculty names to help them track the competition and work on their math skills. There's even a teacher weight tracker worksheet for sale on Teachers Pay Teachers for $9.99, for the purpose of such a competition. For more student-facing activities, there are "Biggest Loser" themed worksheets for teaching and practicing math skills like rate of change.[352]

Workplace wellness initiatives can build community, but once again, leaders must take care to ensure that they are not building community around the toxic idea that thinness is superior. Personalized wellness initiatives that include everyone and are accessible to all take into account that wellness and weight loss are independent factors. Just like we do for students, making messaging as inclusive as possible is key, regardless of our intention. Some schoolwide wellness initiatives can quickly become about the "performance" of health, especially for the fattest among us. In her essay for *This Magazine*, teacher Dani Jansen recalls both her student and teacher experience in a fat body:

> **Quick Tip**
>
> *Help your school frame wellness more holistically around wellness and community, not weight loss.*

As a student, I learned firsthand school was a place where fat kids got bullied. I was called "whale" and "fatty" and once I overheard a friend of my sister's tell her she'd kill herself if she ever got as fat as me. I was maybe a size 12 or 14 at the time. As a teacher, I learned that fatphobia, whether institutionalized or personal, is baked into the school experience.[246]

Jansen mentions that fatphobia takes two forms – the institutional and the interpersonal. Up to now, we've seen some of the ways that anti-fat bias is systemic and, in many cases, glaringly harmful. But many underestimate the personal ways that fatphobia lives in our casual conversations and how deeply harmful it can be. As Jansen points out, what happens in these personal interactions like the one she described is that it translates to folks telling those in fat bodies (with and without saying it) that they would do anything not to be like them, even if it means self-harm or death.[246]

What we know about shame as a motivator, especially when discussing weight loss, is that it doesn't work. In fact, weight stigma and shame may end up costing insurance companies more in the long run for mental and physical healthcare claims; increased weight stigma leads to poorer physical health outcomes, including all-cause mortality.[353] Often, fat peoples' response to this kind of sentiment, whether it's pointed or not, is to become the "good fatty"; performing acts of thinness to "prove" they're trying to behave in ways that would otherwise yield health, like eating salads, low carb, intermittent fasting, going to the gym, skipping dessert, or defensively touting perfect bloodwork (a reflex rooted in ableism and healthism, too).

Fat people do not need to be trying to lose weight to be worthy of promotions, raises, and dignity. The truth is, fat people do not owe anyone their bill of health to receive basic respect, at school or otherwise. Wellness programs focused on weight turn the health of the workplace, the healthcare costs spent by a company, and the insurance coverage they do or don't pay for a matter of employees' personal responsibility. We hear the same language embedded into "work-life balance," which renders working too much the fault of the employee, and not the fault of the workplace for assigning too many tasks, not hiring enough staff, and relying on people to cover, and placing unrealistic expectations and outcomes on those who already work the most. Aubrey Gordon states: "Workplace wellness programs may seem harmless, or even altruistic, aimed at cutting costs and improving employees' health. But data on the effectiveness of workplace wellness programs is largely imperfect and conflicting." In a 2019 study of over 32,000 employees at over 160 workplaces, those who participated in a wellness program reported "significantly greater rates of some positive health behaviors compared with those who were not exposed," but, they reported, "there were no significant effects on clinical measures of health, healthcare spending and utilization, or employment outcomes after 18 months."[347] Many insurance plans have begun to cover weight loss drugs like Ozempic and Wegovy, which help lower blood sugar in people with type 2 diabetes. But even those without diabetes are using it for weight loss, and it has become somewhat synonymous with health promotion. Without insurance, these drugs can cost up to $1,300 a month to acquire.[354] They have become more ubiquitous in the past two years, going from lack of FDA approval to seemingly unending commercials and ads promoting their use. The coverage of weight loss drugs by insurance also, in turn, makes diet talk more ubiquitous in the workplace. As long as we societally cast rapid weight loss in a positive light, the diet culture "bragging rights" that come with it will remain in our faculty rooms.

In many cases, insurance policies use BMI to determine coverage, due in part to the Obama administration's focus on wellness by linking it to health. Mrs. Obama's *Let's Move!* campaign had some of these direct implications for the landmark Affordable Care Act, colloquially known as Obamacare. According to an article by Anna Louise Pickens, "As a result of the Affordable Care Act, employers can charge employees an extra 30 percent of the cost of their health care plans if they don't meet wellness or BMI guidelines."[229] This is a ten point increase from 2006, in which HIPAA allowed a 20 percent increase for those who did not meet BMI guidelines. This is, simply, no-so-thinly-veiled weight discrimination. Also mentioned in the article is a 2015 case, in which a Florida-based first-grade teacher named Tracy Raymond made national news after her job notified her that her premiums would increase by as much as $50 a month if she didn't lose weight.[349] These penalties remained in effect despite little evidence that they reduced healthcare costs. According to Abby Ellin in *Observer*: "Most wellness programs, roughly a six billion dollar a year industry, typically target exercise habits and drug and alcohol use. But those behaviors, experts point out, are *changeable*, whereas size is more complex." In the article, she quotes former chair of the Obesity Action Coalition Ted Kyle, who says

> BMI is a calculation based on two factors—height and weight. We have it drummed into us that weight is under our control. But as a matter of fact, weight is not under your control more than height is. So, how absurd would it be if an employer started setting goals for how tall you could be?[349]

Unfortunately, that's not even the most absurd thing someone has said about teachers and healthcare. In a 2008 piece for Thomas B. Fordham Institute, President Michael Petrilli says that "teacher obesity" is a rising problem in education, in large part because teachers pay "little or nothing for health insurance" thanks to "overgenerous collective bargaining agreements" that make us "oblivious to the cost of healthcare." Their solution? Stop giving teachers "free healthcare," and they will eat less McDonald's. Maybe, Petrulli says, they could start paying into "Weight Watchers style programs on school grounds" instead.[355]

On a personal note, if it were not for the healthcare I receive through my job as a public school teacher, and for the Family Medical Leave Act (FMLA) and for fiercely compassionate administrators, I would not have recovered from the thyroid cancer I was diagnosed with at age 30 during my tenure year.

My weight had ballooned to the highest it had ever been, and I didn't find it curious as a fact on its own until the pieces aligned at my annual physical over the summer. My primary care physician, Kayla, a literal angel on earth, did a "neck check" as is standard, and said abruptly, "ummmm, that feels...enlarged."

The rest of the exam went fine, including my bloodwork which came back normal, and she ordered an ultrasound for my thyroid in case of potential nodules, which are relatively common in the United States.

On the first superintendent's conference day of the year, I got a biopsy of the neck to confirm what was going on with the nodules they found at a cellular level. On the first day of school, my results came back as soon as I pulled into my driveway – *positive for malignant cells – papillary carcinoma*. It made sense why I gained so much weight, but still, I had attributed my feeling easily winded to the weight gain as well (thanks, internalized weight stigma). It was mostly due, actually, to the tumor encasing my thyroid gland and spreading to my neck, which had reached around six centimeters when it was captured on a CT scan later that September.

I am beyond grateful to be cancer-free today, but know that any doctor who hadn't been thorough and told me to just lose weight might have stalled the process of finding out that I had a tumor, and related Hashimoto's thyroiditis, which slows metabolism – and placed the personal responsibility of my fatness solely on my weight. I have also been in remission from an eating disorder for nearly three years. As it turned out, my body became fatter as a way of telling me something was wrong. In a situation such as this, everyone in a society mired by diet culture expects a health scare to be a "scared straight" experience – one that will make a person with an unruly body like mine eat only kale, drink only water, and never eat sugar again for the rest of my life. But this experience taught me that I also will never stop fighting for the dignity, respect, and freedom of larger bodied people, whether or not I remain one myself.

RUN IT BACK – Reflecting on Your Practice

♦ *How do I see professionalism in the field of education, and what, if at all, does my perception of professionalism have to do with size or weight?*

◆ *In what ways is "wellness" at work centered around weight or weight loss? How can I help make a change in the tone of these programs at my school?*

◆ *What explicit or implicit messaging is hiding in the dialogue I have with colleagues? What are some ways I can help shift the conversation?*

9

We're All in This Together
Collaborating for Change

In bringing together all the ideas outlined in this book, I hope one thing is clear: we are all in this together.

But another thing is also true: that simply knowing is not enough to get us out of diet culture. As Dr. Keanga-Yamahatta Taylor says, "we cannot educate ourselves out of structures; inaction, not ignorance, is the root of inequality."[20] This book has equipped you with new ways of thinking or seeing weight bias, weight stigma, size discrimination, and healthism – as well as how it interacts with structures like racism, ableism, xenophobia, classism, and gender bias. Knowing is the first step. In order to lessen the hold that diet culture has on our schools, and our society, we must act our way out of these harms that we do to ourselves, our colleagues, and our students.

After many professional development sessions I've facilitated, I've received feedback to the tune of "now that you've shown me, I can't unsee it," and that's exactly what I could hope for in this work. But once we see it, it is our responsibility to disrupt, challenge, and shift anti-fat bias to create schools where love, justice, weight neutrality, and body liberation are the norm.

DOI: 10.4324/9781003534143-12

I've heard so many times and in so many places that public education is the most radical idea that America has ever had. But there are still ways in which public education is oppressive, mired in corporate profit and interest, and teaching children implicitly and explicitly that some bodies, and the people who inhabit them, matter more than others. Weight bias is just one way that happens. And knowing that means knowing that we have a lot of work to do. But understanding that these are structures; not individual problems that will go away if we are just kind enough, just loving enough, just compassionate enough; is also the work ahead of us. We cannot kindness poster our way out of fatphobia. We must act to shift and change it through culture shifts, expectations, and explicit everyday moves like the ones outlined here in this book.

The tough work ahead is knowing that people – your colleagues, your students, and their caregivers – may resist the idea that we can decouple weight from health. Diet culture, after all, is part of the air we breathe. Meeting people where they are in diet land may feel daunting, counterintuitive, and like taking steps back. But nobody has to do the work perfectly at all times. Perfectionism is a tool of diet culture and white supremacy culture, and doesn't help the goal of a body-liberated school environment progress. Each person in a school environment is a leader – teachers lead classrooms, administrators lead buildings and districts, coaches lead teachers – and the step that comes after gaining knowledge is understanding that knowing that there is harm being done in the world, we have a responsibility to change it. The third step is making a commitment to using that knowledge to end the harm that we know and can't "unsee."

Even if everyone is not yet on board with ending diet culture in school, the message should always be: we are in this together. Nobody will judge you for where you are in the process. But we are moving ahead with creating a space where all bodies are welcome, seen, safe, and valued, regardless of whether we are all ready and regardless of whether our "readiness" looks the same. Because if we wait until we are ready, we allow harm to continue in the name of our anxieties about "getting it right" or "doing things perfectly." And trust me – that's what my eating disorder sounded like. But in this work, perfectionism serves as an avoidance strategy that places the comfort of the most privileged and powerful over the visceral feelings of the harm done to those who have the least privilege and power – in this case, our fat colleagues, students, and community members – and that only aims to perpetuate it so that nothing materially changes. Here are a few ways that perfectionism, delay, or avoidance might show up in this work:

- ◆ **The urge to personalize or individuate (avoidance):** In diet culture, shifting the focus both onto and off of ourselves as a way of perpetuating anti-fat bias is a common way that it persists. For example, saying things like "You're so brave for wearing that. I could never!" or "I really just don't feel like that extra weight is good for me, but if you're happy that way, that's cool" implies that we want to maintain some distance from fatness or proximity to people reading them as fat, while other people cannot. It suggests that something is wrong with existing in a fat body, and ignores that we cannot stand alone inside of systems that are harming those we work with, teach, or care about. Alongside the urge to personalize is a form of denial that weight discrimination, like all forms of discrimination, is a systemic issue.
- ◆ **Fixed or rigid views of health science (avoidance):** Science changes all the time because it's supposed to. And that means, when we find new information, we're supposed to move differently with it. A lot of what we know about dieting has less to do with health than it does with marketing, profit, and money, but media marketing and more have packaged it to us as objective truth. We now know, for example, that weight stigma can be more damaging to health than "excess" weight itself, and that the factors that determine our weight are approximately seventy percent genetic and thirty percent actionable. Our students and colleagues who face anti-fat bias on a

daily basis can't afford to cling to these old ways of being, because they are actively harming them. "If we do what we've always done, we will get what we've always got."

♦ **Denying ownership because of content area or role in a school (delaying and avoiding):** As we've covered before in the book, it doesn't matter if you don't teach health or physical education – creating safe, equitable school environments is everybody's job. That includes the school clerical staff, the nurses, the teachers, the administrators, campus supervisors, paraprofessionals, custodial staff, community volunteers, and culinary specialists. It also includes anyone invited into schools to consult, coach, or observe. Justice is everyone's job, regardless of whether you are directly handling the content where these conversations typically happen as part of your role in a school. The responsibility to learn and act is on all of us, and none of us is exempt from this work.

♦ **Not wanting to "offend" anyone (perfectionism):** This is the most common one when it comes to the first step of even just using "fat" as a descriptive term and decoupling it from its ubiquity as a pejorative, demeaning term. Many of the adults in a school setting have grown up hearing this word in a mean way, and thus, they resist saying it and instead opt for euphemisms like "big boned" or "husky," but these words do nothing to rescue the word "fat" from its status. It also, again, serves to quieten the experiences of fat people rather than normalize them, adding to stigma; there is nothing inherently immoral, wrong, or bad about being in a fat body, and naming the experience is a way that we make that more true for the kids, colleagues, and loved ones living in a fat body. Just say fat.

♦ **Fear of being "called out" (avoidance, perfectionism):** It can be really scary to get it wrong – but when we're dealing with the human experience, it's part of the process. Inevitably, we will all say something we wish we hadn't, and we can't account for where everyone is on their journey. And certainly, we can't expect every situation to be perfectly free from harm every time. We are all learning. But we can't let our fear of others holding us accountable for when we do, inevitably, get it wrong, prevent us from trying to reduce harm. If we are aiming our compass in the direction of reducing the ways that anti-fat bias, racism, sexism, and other oppressions hurt people, including ourselves – we are doing the right thing. Take feedback. Move on with it. And move differently next time. Doing the right thing has to be more important than always, unfailingly, doing it right.

That's not to say that our impact doesn't matter at all. When we intend to do well, missing the mark can happen, and in this case, it often happens at other people's expense. The joke you made to break the ice might have just been better off as silence. Often, when we say the wrong thing, it's because we are leading with discomfort and anxiety. Fatphobic language often fills the air space as a desire to connect with others over what we think or assume we have in common. What else can you add to your desire for connection with others?

The less we avoid, deny, delay, and aim for perfection, the sooner we can get to work. And when we stop derailing the progress of equity in general, the sooner the felt sense of belonging will happen for the very people this work is meant to help heal in our learning spaces. This is a marathon, not a sprint. It's a multi-part harmony, not a solo. We cannot begin unlearning, pausing, and remixing the ways that we show up to do better by our communities, unless we have each other.

THE LAST VERSE: Reflecting on Your Practice

◆ *How do you plan to move differently in your teaching, as it relates to anti-fat bias and size inclusivity?*

◆ *What, for you, feels clearer or more harmonious? What still feels challenging or discordant?*

◆ *Who do you want to join you on this work the most?*

References

1. Gordon, A. (2021, March 29). *I'm a Fat Activist: Here's Why I Don't Use the Word "Fatphobia."* SELF. https://www.self.com/story/fat-activist-fatphobia

2. Gordon, A. (2023). *You Just Need to Lose Weight* (p. xxi). Beacon Press.

3. Pickett, A. C., & Cunningham, G. B. (2017). Physical Activity for Every Body: A Model for Managing Weight Stigma and Creating Body-Inclusive Spaces. *Quest, 69*, 19–36.

4. Forbes, M. (2021). *Body Happy Kids: How to Help Children and Teens Love the Skin They're In*. Vermilion.

5. Bauer, K. W., Yang, Y. W., & Austin, S. B. (2004). "How Can We Stay Healthy When You're Throwing All of This in Front of Us?" Findings from Focus Groups and Interviews in Middle Schools on Environmental Influences on Nutrition and Physical Activity. *Health Education & Behavior, 31*(1), 34–46. https://www.jstor.org/stable/45055142

6. Nerenberg, J. (2020). *Divergent Mind: Thriving in a World that Wasn't Designed for You*. HarperOne.

7. Sole-Smith, V. (2022, July 26). *What Thin Kids Need to Learn about Fatphobia*. Burnt Toast by Virginia Sole-Smith. https://virginiasolesmith.substack.com/p/thin-kids-fatphobia

8. Richardson, S. A., Goodman, N., Hastorf, A. H., & Dornbusch, S. M. (1961). Cultural Uniformity in Reaction to Physical Disabilities. *American Sociological Review, 26*, 241–247.

9. Tutt, P. (2022, February 25). *Weight Bias Hurts Kids, and We're Not Talking about It*. Edutopia. https://www.edutopia.org/article/weight-bias-hurts-kids-and-were-not-talking-about-it

10. Puhl, R. M., Luedicke, J., & Heuer, C. (2011, November). Weight-Based Victimization Toward Overweight Adolescents: Observations and Reactions of Peers. *Journal of School Health, 81*(11), 696–703. https://doi.org/10.1111/j.1746-1561.2011.00646.x

11. Puhl, R., Luedicke, J., & King, K. M. (2015). Combating Weight-Based Bullying in Schools: Is There Public Support for the Use of Litigation?

Journal of School Health, 85(6), 372–381. https://doi.org/10.1111/josh.12264

12. Lessard, L. M., & Lawrence, S. E. (2022). Weight-Based Disparities in Youth Mental Health: Scope, Social Underpinnings, and Policy Implications. *Policy Insights from the Behavioral and Brain Sciences, 9*(1), 49–56. https://doi.org/10.1177/23727322211068018

13. Tovar, V. (2018). *You Have the Right to Remain Fat.* Melville House Uk.

14. Love, B. (2019). *We Want to Do More Than Survive: Abolitionist Teaching and the Pursuit of Educational Freedom.* Beacon.

15. Trine University. (n.d.). *The Effect that Weight Loss and Weight Classes Have on a Wrestler.* https://www.trine.edu/academics/centers/center-for-sports-studies/blog/2021/the_affect_that_weight_loss_and_weight_classes_have_on_a_wrestler.aspx

16. Strings, S. (2019). *Fearing the Black Body: The Racial Origins of Fatphobia.* New York University Press.

17. Gordon, A. (2020). *What We Don't Talk about When We Talk about Fat.* Beacon Press.

18. Sole-Smith, V. (2023). *Fat Talk: Parenting in the Age of Diet Culture.* Bonnier Books UK.

19. Wann, M. (1998). *Fat! So?: Because You Don't Have to Apologize for Your Size!* (p. 208). Ten Speed Press.

20. Hunger, J. M., & Tomiyama, A. J. (2014). Weight Labeling and Obesity: A Longitudinal Study of Girls Aged 10 to 19 Years. *JAMA Pediatrics, 168*(6), 579–580. https://doi.org/10.1001/jamapediatrics.2014.122

21. Angell, M., & Kassirer, J. P. (1998). Alternative Medicine—The Risks of Untested and Unregulated Remedies. *The New England Journal of Medicine, 339*(12), 839–841. https://doi.org/10.1056/NEJM199809173391210

22. Gordon, A. (2019, September 30). *What I Learned as an 11 Year Old in Weight Watchers.* SELF. https://www.self.com/story/kid-in-weight-watchers

23. Lampard, A. M., MacLehose, R. F., Eisenberg, M. E., Neumark-Sztainer, D., & Davison, K. K. (2014). Weight-Related Teasing in the School Environment: Associations with Psychosocial Health and Weight Control Practices among Adolescent Boys and Girls. *Journal of Youth and Adolescence, 43*(10), 1770–1780. https://doi.org/10.1007/s10964-013-0086-3

24. Weinstock, J., & Krehbiel, M. (2009). Fat Youth as Targets for Bullying. In E. Rothblum & S. Solovay (Eds.), *The Fat Studies Reader*. NYU Press, pp. 120–126.

25. Muhammad, G. (2023). *Unearthing Joy: A Guide to Culturally and Historically Responsive Teaching and Learning*. Scholastic Professional.

26. Isono, M., Watkins, P. L., & Lian, L. E. (2023). Bon Bon Fatty Girl: A Qualitative Exploration of Weight Bias in Singapore. In E. Rothblum & S. Solovay (Eds.), *The Fat Studies Reader*. NYU Press, pp. 127–138.

27. Puhl, R. M., Lessard, L. M., Pearl, R. L., Grupski, A., & Foster, G. D. (2021). Policies to Address Weight Discrimination and Bullying: Perspectives of Adults Engaged in Weight Management from Six Nations. *Obesity*, *29*(11), 1787–1798. https://doi.org/10.1002/oby.23275

28. New York State Education Department. (2012). *The Dignity for All Students Act (DASA)*. New York State Education Department. https://www.nysed.gov/content/dignity-all-students-act-dasa

29. New York State Department of Health. (2024, February). *Student Weight Status Data*. https://www.health.ny.gov/prevention/obesity/statistics_and_impact/student_weight_status_data.htm

30. Himmelstein, M. S., Puhl, R. M., & Watson, R. J. (2019). Weight-Based Victimization, Eating Behaviors, and Weight-Related Health in Sexual and Gender Minority Adolescents. *Appetite*, *141*, 104321. https://doi.org/10.1016/j.appet.2019.104321

31. Harvey, R. (2019, March 28). *Eating Disorders Do Not Discriminate: Trans Teens Face Greater Risk*. Penn Medicine. https://www.pennmedicine.org/news/news-blog/2019/march/eating-disorders-do-not-discriminate-trans-teens-face-greater-risk

32. Manfredi, A. (2019). *The (other) F Word: A Celebration of the Fat & Fierce*. Amulet Books, An Imprint of Abrams.

33. ABC News. (2009, April 1). *Teen Commits Suicide Due to Bullying: Parents Sue School for Son's Death*. ABC News. https://abcnews.go.com/Health/MindMoodNews/story?id=7228335

34. Campos, P. F. (2004). *The Obesity Myth: Why America's Obsession with Weight Is Hazardous to Your Health*. Gotham Books.

35. Associated Press. (1997, October 2). *Teenager Takes Overdose after Suffering Years of Taunts*. Sarasota Herald Tribune. https://news.google.com/newspapers?id=sLMcAAAAIBAJ&pg=6852

36. van den Berg, P., Neumark-Sztainer, D., Eisenberg, M. E., & Haines, J. (2008). Racial/Ethnic Differences in Weight-related Teasing in Adolescents. *Obesity, 16,* S3–S10. https://doi.org/10.1038/oby.2008.445

37. ACLU Ohio. (2016, January 8). *Black Children Are Children: Tamir Rice and the Adultification of Black Bodies.* ACLU of Ohio. https://www.acluohio.org/en/news/black-children-are-children-tamir-rice-and-adultification-black-bodies

38. Asare, J. G. (2021). *How the Adultification Bias Contributes to Black Trauma.* Forbes. https://www.forbes.com/sites/janicegassam/2021/04/22/how-the-adultification-bias-contributes-to-black-trauma/

39. Associated Press. (2014, November 25). *Darren Wilson: "I felt like a 5-year-old holding onto Hulk Hogan."* https://www.cbsnews.com/news/ferguson-decision-darren-wilson-said-he-felt-like-a-5-year-old-holding-onto-hulk-hogan/

40. Mercedes, M. (2020). Public Health's Power Neutral, Fatphobic Obsession with "Food Deserts." *Marquisele Mercedes.* https://www.marquiselemercedes.com/read/food-deserts

41. Dian, M., & Triventi, M. (2021). The Weight of School Grades: Evidence of Biased Teachers' Evaluations against Overweight Students in Germany. *PLOS ONE, 16*(2), e0245972. https://doi.org/10.1371/journal.pone.0245972

42. Finn, K. E., Seymour, C. M., & Phillips, A. E. (2019). Weight Bias and Grading among Middle and High School Teachers. *British Journal of Educational Psychology, 90*(3), 635–647. https://doi.org/10.1111/bjep.12322

43. Hetrick, A., & Attig, D. (2006). Sitting Pretty: Fat Bodies, Classroom Desks & Academic Excess. In E. Rothblum & S. Solovay (Eds.), *The Fat Studies Reader.* NYU Press, pp. 197–204.

44. Jones, S. (2019, November 25). *Ending Curriculum Violence.* Learning for Justice. https://www.learningforjustice.org/magazine/spring-2020/ending-curriculum-violence

45. Lerner, R. M., & Gellert, E. (1969). Body Build Identification, Preference, and Aversion in Children. *Developmental Psychology, 1*(5), 456–462. https://doi.org/10.1037/h0027966

46. Staffieri, J. R. (1972). Body Build and Behavioral Expectancies in Young Females. *Developmental Psychology, 6*(1), 125–127. https://doi.org/10.1037/h0032211

47. Harriger, J. A., & Trammell, J. P. (2021). First Do No Harm: Measuring Weight Bias Beliefs in Preschool-Age Children. *Body Image, 40,* 176–181.

48. Holub, S. C. (2008). Individual Differences in the Ant-Fat Attitudes of Preschool-Children: The Importance of Perceived Body Size. *Body Image*, *5*, 317–321. https://doi.org/10.1016/J.bodyim.2008.03.003

49. Musher-Eizenman, D. R. (2004). Body Size Stigmatization in Preschool Children: The Role of Control Attributions. *Journal of Pediatric Psychology*, *29*(8), 613–620. https://doi.org/10.1093/jpepsy/jsh063

50. Worobey, J., & Worobey, H. S. (2014). Body-Size Stigmatization by Preschool Girls: In a Doll's World, It Is Good to Be "Barbie". *Body Image*, *11*(2), 171–174. https://doi.org/10.1016/j.bodyim.2013.12.001

51. Cramer, P., & Steinwert, T. (1998). Thin Is Good, Fat Is Bad: How Early Does It Begin? *Journal of Applied Developmental Psychology*, *19*(3), 429–451. https://doi.org/10.1016/S0193-3973(99)80049-5

52. Marx, J. M., Kiefner-Burmeister, A., Roberts, L. T., & Musher-Eizenman, D. R. (2019). Nothing Alien about It: A Comparison of Weight Bias in Preschool-Aged Children's Ratings of Non-Human Cartoons and Human Figures. *Obesity Research & Clinical Practice*, *13*(5), 435–439. https://doi.org/10.1016/j.orcp.2019.09.002

53. Hafner, M. L. (2018). *The Joy of Movement: Lesson Plans and Large-motor Activities for Preschoolers*. Redleaf Press.

54. Hartmann, J. (2019). Jack Hartmann Kids Music Channel [YouTube Video]. *YouTube*. https://www.youtube.com/user/JackHartmann

55. Amlund, D. (2020, May 19). *Will Fatphobia Cause Eugenics?* Konfront. https://konfront.dk/will-fatphobia-cause-eugenics/

56. Lessard, L. M., & Puhl, R. M. (2021). Adolescents' Exposure to and Experiences of Weight Stigma During the COVID-19 Pandemic. *Journal of Pediatric Psychology*, *46*(8), 950–959. https://doi.org/10.1093/jpepsy/jsab071

57. Butler-Wall, K. (2015). Risky Measures: Digital Technologies and the Governance of Child Obesity. *WSQ: Women's Studies Quarterly*, *43*(1), 228–245. https://muse.jhu.edu/article/581529

58. Lupton, D. (2012). *Fat*. London: Routledge.

59. Blakemore, S.-J., & Mills, K. L. (2014). Is Adolescence a Sensitive Period for Sociocultural Processing? *Annual Review of Psychology*, *65*, 187–207. https://doi.org/10.1146/annurev-psych-010213-115202

60. Pearl, R. L. (2020). Weight Stigma and the "Quarantine-15." *Obesity*, *28*(7), 1180–1181. https://doi.org/10.1002/oby.22850

61. Gowers, S. G., & Shore, A. (2001). Development of Weight and Shape Concerns in the Aetiology of Eating Disorders. *British Journal of Psychiatry*, *179*(3), 236–242. https://doi.org/10.1192/bjp.179.3.236

62. Hanson, O. (2023, September 12). *Is Your Kid Learning Diet Culture at School?* Parenting Without Diet Culture. https://oonahanson.substack.com/p/is-your-kid-learning-diet-culture

63. Beckwith, S., Cooper, M., Goesch, H., MacKinnon, G., Anderson, D., & Stang, J. (2017). *Nutrition Education in America's Schools: A Policy Brief.* Association of State Public Health Nutritionists. https://asphn.org/wp-content/uploads/2017/10/2016-Nutrition-Education-in-Americas-Schools.pdf

64. O'Connor, C. [@justteachingela]. (2022, 26 September). *Please stop assigning food diaries to students: please.* Twitter (X).

65. Hanson, O. (2024, May 25). *This Film Is Still Shown to Students as If It Were Simply a Presentation of Nutrition Facts: Food Documentaries—Especially Without Any Attention to Media Literacy and Critical Thinking—Harm Adolescents, Who Are Already Vulnerable to Eating Disorders and Negative Body Image.* https://x.com/OonaHanson/status/1794443906098290798

66. Editorial Board. (2007, November 3). *Carmona: Obesity is "the terror within."* Arizona Daily Star. https://tucson.com/news/science/carmona-obesity-is-the-terror-within/article_62567ec3-0647-5074-b19d-7b7f8562cd31.html

67. Sarner, L. (2024, May 24). *Morgan Spurlock Dead: "Super Size Me" Filmmaker Dies at 53.* New York Post. https://nypost.com/2024/05/24/entertainment/morgan-spurlock-dead-super-size-me-filmmaker-dies-at-53/

68. Hanson, O. (2024, June 5). *Food Films Are Not Nutrition Education.* Parenting Without Diet Culture. https://oonahanson.substack.com/p/food-films-are-not-nutrition-education

69. Center for Disease Control. (2024, May 14). *Social Determinants of Health.* Public Health Professionals Gateway. https://www.cdc.gov/public-health-gateway/php/about/social-determinants-of-health.html

70. Johnson, C. (2024). *What health actually includes.* Instagram.

71. Poulain, M., Herm, A., & Pes, G. (2013). The Blue Zones: Areas of Exceptional Longevity around the World. *Vienna Yearbook of Population Research, 11*, 87–108. https://www.jstor.org/stable/43050798

72. Petrzela, N. M. (2022, September 24). *Why American Kids Grow Up Hating Exercise.* Slate. https://slate.com/human-interest/2022/09/history-physical-education-kids-sports-inclusive-exercise.html

73. Lucibello, K. M., Sabiston, C. M., Pila, E., & Arbour-Nicitopoulos, K. (2023). An Integrative Model of Weight Stigma, Body Image, and Physical Activity in Adolescents. *Body Image*, *45*, 1–10. https://doi.org/10.1016/j.bodyim.2023.01.003

74. Bauer, K. W., Yang, Y. W., & Austin, S. B. (2004). "How Can We Stay Healthy When You're Throwing All of This in Front of Us?" Findings From Focus Groups and Interviews in Middle Schools on Environmental Influences on Nutrition and Physical Activity. *Health Education & Behavior*, *31*(1), 34–46. https://www.jstor.org/stable/45055142

75. Bacon, L., & Aphramor, L. (2014). *Body Respect: What Conventional Health Books Get Wrong, Leave Out, and Just Plain Fail to Understand about Weight*. Benbella Books.

76. Spell, C. S. (2016, November 4). *There's No Sugar-Coating It: All Calories Are Not Created Equal*. Harvard Health Blog. https://www.health.harvard.edu/blog/theres-no-sugar-coating-it-all-calories-are-not-created-equal-2016110410602

77. CDC. (2023, May 8). *Facts about Suicide*. Centers for Disease Control and Prevention. https://www.cdc.gov/suicide/facts/index.html

78. Alli, R. A. (Ed.). (2023, April 25). *What to Know about Dieting and Mental Health in Teens*. WebMD. https://www.webmd.com/children/what-to-know-about-dieting-and-mental-health-in-teens

79. Levinson, C. A., Hunt, R. A., Christian, C., Williams, B. M., Keshishian, A. C., Vanzhula, I. A., & Ralph-Nearman, C. (2022). Longitudinal Group and Individual Networks of Eating Disorder Symptoms in Individuals Diagnosed with an Eating Disorder. *Journal of Psychopathology and Clinical Science, 131*(1), 58. https://doi.org/10.1037/abn0000727

80. MHA National. (2024). *Eating Disorders and Youth*. Mental Health America. https://www.mhanational.org/eating-disorders-and-youth

81. Harrison, C. (2018, December). *The Truth about High Weight Anorexia with Erin Harrop* (No. 178) [Podcast]. Food Psych. https://christyharrison.com/foodpsych/6/the-truth-about-atypical-anorexia-with-erin-harrop

82. Hawgood, A. (2022, March 5). What Is "Bigorexia"? *The New York Times*. https://www.nytimes.com/2022/03/05/style/teen-bodybuilding-bigorexia-tiktok.html

83. Alleva, J. M., Sheeran, P., Webb, T. L., Martijn, C., & Miles, E. (2015). A Meta-Analytic Review of Stand-Alone Interventions to Improve Body Image. *PLoS One, 10*(9), e0139177. https://doi.org/10.1371/journal.pone.0139177

84. Natterson, C., & Kroll Bennett, V. (2023, November 14). Talk to Your Boys (Season 3, Episode 20). *This is so Awkward*. https://podcasts.apple.com/us/podcast/talk-to-your-boys/id1576221880?i=1000725667094

85. Jones, B. (2023, October 10). *Ghrelin and Leptin: Hormones, Hunger, Weight Changes*. Verywell Health. https://www.verywellhealth.com/ghrelin-and-leptin-7970365

86. Sports & Physical Education. (2022, June 28). Kraus – Weber Fitness Test Minimum Muscular Fitness Test. *YouTube*. https://www.youtube.com/watch?v=WUllunADpNU

87. Mukherjee, R., Pandya, P., Baxi, D., & Ramachandran, A. V. (2021). Endocrine Disruptors–"Food" for Thought. *Proceedings of the Zoological Society*, 74(4), 432–442. https://doi.org/10.1007/s12595-021-00414-1

88. Cleveland Clinic. (2022, March 18). *Serotonin*. Cleveland Clinic. https://my.clevelandclinic.org/health/articles/22572-serotonin

89. U.S. Copyright Office. (2025). *U.S. Copyright Office Public Records System*. Copyright.gov; Remitter Portal. https://publicrecords.copyright.gov/search?page_number=1&query=%22presidential%20physical%20fitness%22&field_type=%22keyword%22&records_per_page=10&sort_order=%22asc%22&model=%22%22

90. Wikipedia Contributors. (2024, February 20). *Kraus–Weber Test*. Wikipedia; Wikimedia Foundation. https://en.wikipedia.org/wiki/Kraus%E2%80%93Weber_test#cite_note-4

91. Boyle, R. (1955). The Report that Shocked the President. *Sports Illustrated*, *30–33*, 72–75.

92. Edwards, P. (2015, April 24). *A Brief History of the Bizarre and Sadistic Presidential Fitness Test*. Vox. https://www.vox.com/2015/4/24/8489501/presidential-fitness-test

93. Martin, D. (2011, December 19). *Bonnie Prudden, 97, Dies; Promoted Fitness for TV Generation*. The New York Times. https://www.nytimes.com/2011/12/19/health/bonnie-prudden-dies-at-97-promoted-fitness-for-youths.html

94. Snoddy, A. (March 20, 1975). Never Too Late to Exercise. *The Victoria Advocate*.

95. Prudden, B. (1963). *Teenage Fitness*. Harper & Row.

96. Bonnie Prudden Myotherapy. (n.d.). *Bookstore*. Bonnie Prudden Myotherapy. Retrieved July 7, 2024, from https://bonnieprudden.com/bookstore/

97. Prudden, B. (1972). *Fitness from Six to Twelve*. Harper & Row.

98. Greenleaf, C., & Weiller, K. (2005). Perceptions of Youth Obesity among Physical Educators. *Social Psychology of Education*, 8(4), 407–423. https://doi.org/10.1007/s11218-005-0662-9

99. Carmona Marquez, J., Robles, A. S., Sanchez-Garcia, M., & Garcia Rodriguez, M. P. (2020). Anti-fat Bias in Secondary School Teachers: Are Physical Education Teachers More Biased Than Mathematics Teachers? *European Physical Education Review*, 27(1), 168–184.

100. Old School Trainer. (n.d.). *Could You Survive President JFK's 1960's Phys-Ed Class?* Old School Trainer. https://oldschooltrainer.com/could-you-survive-this-1960s-gym-class/

101. Gordon, S. (1962, January 30). La Sierra High Shows How America Can Get Physically Tough. *Look*, 49–52.

102. John F. Kennedy Presidential Library. (1961). *Council on Youth Fitness: "The Soft American"*. https://www.jfklibrary.org/asset-viewer/archives/jfkpof-094-003#?image_identifier=JFKPOF-094-003-p0009

103. The Cooper Institute. (n.d.). *Youth Initiatives — FitnessGram*. https://www.cooperinstitute.org/youth/fitnessgram

104. Nadworny, E. (2014, November 24). *Tools of the Trade: The Presidential Physical Fitness Test*. NPR. https://www.npr.org/sections/ed/2014/11/24/365716113/tools-of-the-trade-the-presidential-physical-fitness-test

105. Safron, C., & Landi, D. (2021). Beyond the BEEPs: Affect, FitnessGram®, and Diverse Youth. *Sport, Education and Society*, 1–15. https://doi.org/10.1080/13573322.2021.1953978

106. Human Kinetics USA. (n.d.). *Fitnessgram ® Healthy Fitness Zone Standards Frequently Asked Questions*. Retrieved July 7, 2024, from https://www.livingston.org/cms/lib9/NJ01000562/Centricity/Domain/445/newstandardsfaqforprint.pdf

107. Beresini, E. (2024, March 31). *School Fitness Testing Is a Nightmare: Should We Get Rid of It?* Outside Online. https://www.outsideonline.com/health/wellness/school-fitness-testing-backlash-california

108. Fernandez-Balboa, J.-M. (1997). *Critical Postmodernism in Human Movement, Physical Education, and Sport*. SUNY Press.

109. Fitzpatrick, K. (2013). Brown Bodies, Racialisation and Physical Education. *Sport, Education and Society*, 18(2), 135–153. https://doi.org/10.1080/13573322.2011.559221

110. Berg, P., & Kokkonen, M. (2021). Heteronormativity Meets Queering in Physical Education: The Views of PE Teachers and LGBTIQ+ Students. *Physical Education and Sport Pedagogy*, *27*(4), 1–14. https://doi.org/10.1080/17408989.2021.1891213

111. Jet (2001, November 26). Heavy Can Mean Healthy If You're Active, *100*(24), 14. Jet Magazine. Johnson Publishing Company, Chicago, IL.

112. New York City Department of Education. (2023). *DOE Data at a Glance*. NYC Department of Education. https://www.schools.nyc.gov/about-us/reports/doe-data-at-a-glance

113. The Central Park Conservancy. (2018, January 18). *The Story of Seneca Village*. Central Park Conservancy. https://www.centralparknyc.org/articles/seneca-village

114. Williams, K. (2017, December 21). How Lincoln Center Was Built (It Wasn't Pretty). *The New York Times*. https://www.nytimes.com/2017/12/21/nyregion/how-lincoln-center-was-built-it-wasnt-pretty.html

115. New York State Department of Health. (2024). *Student Weight Status Data*. https://www.health.ny.gov/prevention/obesity/statistics_and_impact/student_weight_status_data.htm

116. New York State Department of Health. (2010). *High Need for Chronic Disease Prevention and Management NG Persons with DI in New York State (NYS) Public Health Opportunity Percentage of Elementary School Students*. https://www.health.ny.gov/statistics/prevention/injury_prevention/information_for_action/docs/2019-02_ifa_report.pdf

117. State University of New York at Geneseo. (n.d.). *Information on High Needs School Districts*. SUNY Geneseo. Retrieved July 7, 2024, from https://www.geneseo.edu/noyce/information-high-needs-school-districts

118. New York State Department of Health - Division of Chronic Disease Prevention. (2013). *SWSCR 2010-12 IFA 2, Weight Status Distribution by District*. https://www.health.ny.gov/statistics/prevention/injury_prevention/information_for_action/docs/2013-05_ifa_report.pdf

119. NYC Health. (n.d.). *Information for Health Care Professionals Why Should I Be Aware of NYC FITNESSGRAM?* Retrieved July 7, 2024, from https://www.nyc.gov/assets/doh/downloads/pdf/csi/csi-nycfg-faq.pdf

120. Let's Move. (2010). *Learn the Facts*. Archives.gov. https://letsmove.obamawhitehouse.archives.gov/learn-facts/epidemic-childhood-obesity

121. Guthman, J. (2013). Too Much Food and Too Little Sidewalk? Problematizing the Obesogenic Environment Thesis. *Environment and Planning A: Economy and Space, 45*(1), 142–158. https://doi.org/10.1068/a45130

122. Azzarito, L. (2016). "Permission to Speak": A Postcolonial View on Racialized Bodies and PE in the Current Context of Globalization. *Research Quarterly for Exercise and Sport, 87*(2), 141–150. https://doi.org/10.1080/02701367.2016.1166474

123. NYC Public Schools. (2024). *Physical Education.* Web. https://www.schools.nyc.gov/learning/subjects/physical-education

124. Madsen, K. A., Thompson, H. R., Linchey, J., Ritchie, L. D., Gupta, S., Neumark-Sztainer, D., Crawford, P. B., McCulloch, C. E., & Ibarra-Castro, A. (2020). Effect of School-Based Body Mass Index Reporting in California Public Schools: A Randomized Clinical Trial. *JAMA Pediatrics, 175*(3), 251–259. https://doi.org/10.1001/jamapediatrics.2020.4768

125. Center for Disease Control. (2019). *Body Mass Index (BMI) Measurement in Schools.* CDC Healthy Schools. https://www.cdc.gov/healthyschools/obesity/bmi/BMI_measurement_schools.htm

126. Campos, P. (2004). *The Obesity Myth: Why America's Obsession with Weight Is Hazardous to Your Health.* Gotham Books.

127. Ehlert, C., Marston, R., Fontana, F., & Waldron, J. (2015). Weight Bias in Schools and How Physical Educators Can Assist in Its Demise - ProQuest. *Physical Educator, 72*(3), 403–412. ProQuest. https://www.proquest.com/scholarly-journals/weight-bias-schools-how-physical-educators-can/docview/1722191697/se-2?accountid=34782

128. Bacon, L. (2010). *Health at Every Size: The Surprising Truth about Your Weight.* Benbella Books.

129. The Association for Size Diversity and Health. (2024). *The Health at Every Size® (HAES®) Principles.* ASDAH. https://asdah.org/haes/

130. Music, M. (2025). *Dr Oz Mocked for Insisting It's Americans' "Patriotic Duty" to Stay Healthy: "Cutting Medicare Is Unpatriotic."* MSN. https://www.msn.com/en-us/politics/government/dr-oz-mocked-for-insisting-it-s-americans-patriotic-duty-to-stay-healthy-cutting-medicare-is-unpatriotic/ar-AA1EushP

131. Boero, N. (2006). All the News that's Fat to Print: The American "Obesity Epidemic" and the Media. *Qualitative Sociology, 30*(1), 41–60. https://doi.org/10.1007/s11133-006-9010-4

132. Boudreau, C., & Bottemiller Evich, H. (2019). *How Washington Keeps America Sick and Fat*. POLITICO. https://www.politico.com/news/agenda/2019/11/04/why-we-dont-know-what-to-eat-060299

133. Raikar, S. P. (2023, April 26). *Food Pyramid*. Britannica. https://www.britannica.com/science/food-pyramid

134. Freuman, T. D. (2020). *Who Actually Needs a 2,000-Calorie Diet?* US News & World Report; U.S. News & World Report. https://health.usnews.com/health-news/blogs/eat-run/articles/2016-06-14/who-actually-needs-a-2-000-calorie-diet

135. Nestle, M. (2011, August 4). *Why Does the FDA Recommend 2,000 Calories Per Day?* The Atlantic. https://www.theatlantic.com/health/archive/2011/08/why-does-the-fda-recommend-2-000-calories-per-day/243092/

136. Hanson, O. (2023, October 9). *"Healthy Eating" Curriculum Can Do More Harm Than Good*. CNN. https://www.cnn.com/2023/10/09/health/unhealthy-school-nutrition-lessons-wellness/index.html

137. Hanson, O. [oona_hanson]. (2024, July 20). *Summertime food bills*. [Post]. Instagram. LINK.

138. Arnold, T. [@growing.intuitive.eaters]. (2024, January 9). *Have done a few of these lessons* [Video]. Instagram. LINK

139. Arnold, T. [@growing.intuitive.eaters]. (2023, December 11). *What would you add or take away?* [Video]. Instagram. LINK

140. The Edible Schoolyard Project. (2020, October 1). *About Us*. The Edible Schoolyard Project. https://edibleschoolyard.org/about-us

141. Steier, J. (2024). *The Food Babe strikes again...* Instagram. https://www.instagram.com/unbiasedscipod/p/C-kiKyHNfNL/

142. u/cybermage. (2016). *Bob Has Diabetes*. Reddit. https://www.reddit.com/r/funny/comments/4mzao0/bob_has_diabetes/

143. Williams, L. (1995). Stalking the Elusive Healthy Diet. In *Scientific Studies, Seeking the Truth in a Vast Gray Area. New York Times*.

144. Allison, D. B., & Pi-Sunyer, F. X. (1994). Fleshing Out Obesity. *The Sciences*, *34*(3), 38–43. https://doi.org/10.1002/j.2326-1951.1994.tb03166.x

145. Tayag, Y. (2023, May 25). *Ozempic in Teens Is a Mess*. The Atlantic. https://www.theatlantic.com/health/archive/2023/05/ozempic-teen-obesity-treatment-health-promises-risks/674204/

146. Novo Nordisk. (2023, August). *Ozempic® Side Effects Ozempic® (semaglutide) Injection 0.5 mg or 1 mg*. https://www.ozempic.com/how-to-take/side-effects.html

147. Kopf, M., & Nguyen, V. (2024, February 21). *More Teens Are Turning to Weight Loss Drugs*. NBC News. https://www.nbcnews.com/health/kids-health/weight-loss-drugs-teens-ozempic-wegovy-kids-rcna139687

148. Sole-Smith, V., & de la Cretaz, F. (2025, January 30). *Why Is the WNBA Running Weight Loss Ads Now?* Burnt Toast by Virginia Sole-Smith. https://virginiasolesmith.substack.com/p/why-is-the-wnba-running-weight-loss-ads?utm_source=%2Finbox%2Fpaid&utm_medium=reader2

149. DNYUZ. (2025, January 28). *Hims & Hers Is Making a Massive Bet on a Super Bowl Ad This Year*. DNYUZ. https://dnyuz.com/2025/01/28/hims-hers-is-making-a-massive-bet-on-a-super-bowl-ad-this-year/

150. USA Today. (2025). *Hims & Hers Super Bowl Commercial: Ad Draws Ire from Drug Industry*. Ad Meter. https://admeter.usatoday.com/story/sports/ad-meter/2025/02/09/hims-hers-super-bowl-commercial-2025-weight-loss/78253917007/

151. Museum of Science. (2024). *Activity: Golden Ratio*. https://www.mos.org/leonardo/activities/golden-ratio.html#:~:text=The%20golden%20ratio%2C%20also%20known

152. Henley, A. (2016, December 13). *There's a Mathematical Equation That Proves I'm Ugly: Here's How I Learned to Ignore It*. Vox. https://www.vox.com/first-person/2016/12/13/13900086/crouzon-syndrome-golden-ratio-beauty

153. Simone, N. (2020). Nina Simone: An Artist's Duty [YouTube Video]. *YouTube*. https://www.youtube.com/watch?v=99V0mMNf5fo

154. Shearer, C. (2017, February 15). The Thinning of Big Mama. *Oxford American*. New York, NY: The Oxford American Literary Project, Inc. Retrieved January 14, 2024.

155. Hill, C. A. (2016, April 12). Who Owns "Hound Dog"?. *Charles A. Hill Mediation*. Retrieved January 16, 2024.

156. Wikipedia Contributors. (2024, August 15). *Martha Wash*. Wikipedia; Wikimedia Foundation. https://en.wikipedia.org/wiki/Martha_Wash

157. C + C Music Factory. (1990). Gonna Make You Sweat (Everybody Dance Now) (Official HD Video). https://www.youtube.com/watch?v=LaTGrV58wec

158. Kuiper, K. (2018). *Venus of Willendorf Characteristics, Image, & Facts*. Encyclopædia Britannica. https://www.britannica.com/topic/Venus-of-Willendorf

159. Encyclopedia Britannica. (2024). *Sarah Baartman*. Britannica. https://www.britannica.com/biography/Sarah-Baartman

160. Hawthorn, A. (2024, August 9). *Illegal to Be 'Ugly'? The History Behind One of America's Cruelest Laws*. History. https://www.nationalgeographic.com/history/article/history-of-ugly-laws-america-disability

161. PBS. (2018). Why Was It Illegal to Be Ugly? The Origin of Everything (Season 1, Episode 34). https://www.pbs.org/video/why-it-was-illegal-to-be-ugly-c8ps4i/

162. Bates, D. (2015, October 23). *The Real-Life American Horror Story: Freak Show*. Mail Online; Daily Mail. https://www.dailymail.co.uk/news/article-3283496/A-555-pound-woman-ate-10-000-calorie-DAY-diet-Zebraman-bearded-lady-Meet-sideshow-freaks-1930s-went-laughed-overnight-sensations.html

163. Brett, M. (2015). *Freaks of Sideshow and Film: Free Download, Borrow, and Streaming: Internet Archive*. Internet Archive. https://archive.org/details/freaksofsideshow0000bret

164. *The Mermaid Parade*. (n.d.). Coney Island USA. https://www.coneyisland.com/mermaidparade

165. Cillizza, C. (2017). *How Much Did William Howard Taft Actually Weigh?* The Washington Post. https://www.washingtonpost.com/news/the-fix/wp/2017/01/05/how-much-did-william-howard-taft-actually-weigh/

166. Roos, D. (2022, May 31). *The Political Cartoonist Who Helped Lead to "Boss" Tweed's Downfall*. HISTORY. https://www.history.com/news/thomas-nast-boss-tweed-cartoons

167. The Spokesman Review. (1955, August 7). *Dolly Dimples, 555 Pound Fat Lady, Now Turned 225*. Newspapers.com. https://www.newspapers.com/image/568553535/

168. Gerhardt, L. (2020, February 4). *The Rebellious History of the Fat Acceptance Movement*. Center for Discovery. https://centerfordiscovery.com/blog/fat-acceptance-movement/

169. Amanda Martinez Beck. (2022). *More of You*. Broadleaf Books.

170. Wikipedia Contributors. (2025, May 30). *Judy Freespirit*. Wikipedia; Wikimedia Foundation. https://en.wikipedia.org/wiki/Judy_Freespirit

171. Fishman, S. (2024). *Life in the Fat Underground*. Radiancemagazine. com. https://radiancemagazine.com/issues/1998/winter_98/fat_ underground.html

172. Fletcher, D. (2009, July 31). *The Fat-Acceptance Movement*. TIME; nextgen. https://time.com/archive/6914922/the-fat-acceptance-movement/

173. Kazdin, C. (2023). *What's Eating Us*. St. Martin's Essentials.

174. World Health Organization. (2020). *Controlling the Global Obesity Epidemic*. https://www.who.int/activities/controlling-the-global-obesity-epidemic

175. Banville, S. (n.d.). *Breaking News English Lesson: Obesity*. https:// breakingnewsenglish.com/2303/230313-world-obesity.html

176. Muhammad, G. (2023). *Unearthing Joy: A Guide to Culturally and Historically Responsive Teaching and Learning*. Scholastic Professional.

177. Jones, K., & Okun, T. (2001). *White Supremacy Culture from Dismantling Racism: A Workbook For*. Minnesota Historical Society. https://www.thc.texas.gov/public/upload/preserve/museums/ files/White_Supremacy_Culture.pdf

178. Creamer, M., & Swope, E. (2016). *Obesity in Mexico Intermediate-Low Spanish IPA Pack - Digital Resource Download*. Teacher's Discovery. https://teachersdiscovery.com/products/obesity-in-mexico-intermediate-low-spanish-ipa-pack-digital-resource-download?s rsltid=AfmBOoo5PrQ6z646lqvMGJ3BYBdigbBx3lKYnRMb6bD6n C2N_S67n-Nh

179. Alexander, K. (2022). It's a Big Fat Deal: How Schools Teach Contempt for Fat People - and What We Can Do about It. *Rethinking Schools*. https://rethinkingschools.org/articles/its-a-big-fat-deal/.

180. *Shallow Hal* (2001). (n.d.). iMDb. https://www.imdb.com/title/ tt0256380/

181. goop. (2025). *goop Beauty*. Goop.com. https://goop.com/goop-beauty/c/?click_source=nav-3-madebygoop-goopbeauty-shopallgoopbeauty

182. Jennings, R. (2021, January 13). *Can Social Media Ever Be Truly "Body Positive?"* Vox. https://www.vox.com/the-goods/22226997/body-positivity-instagram-tiktok-fatphobia-social-media

183. Psychology Today. (2024). *Parasocial Relationships*. https://www. psychologytoday.com/us/basics/parasocial-relationships

184. BBC. (2022, May 4). Kim Kardashian Criticised over Marilyn Monroe Dress Diet for Met Gala. *BBC News*. https://www.bbc.com/news/entertainment-arts-61318361

185. Kato, B. (2022, January 26). *Kim Kardashian's "Slim-thick" Figure Is "More Harmful for Body Image": Study*. New York Post. https://nypost.com/2022/01/26/kim-kardashians-figure-is-harmful-for-body-image-study/

186. *In the Age of Selfies, America's Love Affair with Lips Is Leading to a Boom in Cosmetic Procedures*. (n.d.). American Society of Plastic Surgeons. https://www.plasticsurgery.org/news/press-releases/in-the-age-of-selfies-americas-love-affair-with-lips-is-leading-to-a-boom-in-cosmetic-procedures

187. Lang, C. (2023, July 28). *Even the Kardashians Can't Keep Up with Their Beauty Ideals*. Time. https://time.com/6298911/kardashians-kylie-jenner-boob-job-beauty-standards/

188. Grace, A. (2024, July 17). *Kylie and Kendall Jenner Spark Ultra-slim "Yacht Shoulders" Trend: "It's Insane."* Yahoo Entertainment. https://www.yahoo.com/entertainment/kylie-kendall-jenner-spark-ultra-144550594.html?rdrctId=adba9f5d-9084-3a15-ae5d-749327c94343

189. Greenfield, B. (2024, July 17). *How "Big Back," "Fatty," and Other "Fatphobic" Slang Is Damaging Your Teen's Mental Health*. Fortune Well; Fortune. https://fortune.com/well/article/big-back-fatty-teen-fat-speak-problem-for-everybody/

190. Centers for Disease Control and Prevention and Bridging the Gap Research Program (2014). *Strategies for Creating Supportive School Nutrition Environments: Update for the 2012-2013 School Year*. U.S. Department of Health and Human Services.

191. Milmo, D., & Paul, K. (2021, September 30). *Facebook Disputes Its Own Research Showing Harmful Effects of Instagram on Teens' Mental Health*. The Guardian. https://www.theguardian.com/technology/2021/sep/29/facebook-hearing-latest-children-impact

192. North, A. (2021, October 18). *The Past, Present, and Future of Body Image in America*. Vox. https://www.vox.com/22697168/body-positivity-image-millennials-gen-z-weight

193. *Eating Disorders and Youth*. (n.d.). Mental Health America. https://www.mhanational.org/eating-disorders-and-youth

194. *The Dangers of Pro-Ana and Pro-Mia*. (2023). Beat Eating Disorders. https://www.beateatingdisorders.org.uk/get-information-

and-support/about-eating-disorders/dangers-of-pro-
ana-and-pro-mia/

195. Clark, O., Lee, M. M., Jingree, M. L., O'Dwyer, E., Yue, Y., Marrero, A.,
Tamez, M., Bhupathiraju, S. N., & Mattei, J. (2021). Weight Stigma
and Social Media: Evidence and Public Health Solutions. *Frontiers
in Nutrition, 8*. https://doi.org/10.3389/fnut.2021.739056

196. Lai, S. (2022, February 24). *How Do We Solve Social Media's Eating
Disorder Problem?* Brookings. https://www.brookings.edu/articles/
how-do-we-solve-social-medias-eating-disorder-problem/

197. Editorial Contributors. (2025, May 2). *How to Talk to Your Kids about
Social Media*. WebMD. https://www.webmd.com/parenting/how-
to-talk-to-kids-about-social-media

198. Falcon, M., & Shoop, S. A. (2003, January 13). *Denise Austin Attacks
Women's Fitness Problems*. USA Today. Retrieved September 7, 2007.

199. *Denise Austin*. (n.d.). https://www.deniseaustin.com/

200. *The Biggest Loser (American TV series)*. (2022, August 7). Wikipedia.
https://en.wikipedia.org/wiki/The_Biggest_Loser_(American_
TV_series)

201. Wyatt, E. (2009, November 25). *On 'The Biggest Loser,' Health Can
Take Back Seat"*. The New York Times. Retrieved November 26, 2009.

202. Hosie, R. (2022, December 7). *What Jillian Michaels Eats in a Day to
Stay Fit and Support Her Metabolism*. Business Insider Africa. https://
africa.businessinsider.com/health/what-jillian-michaels-eats-in-a-
day-to-stay-fit-and-support-her-metabolism/9jpm3b6

203 Sears, B. (2016, May 10). *Gaining It Back: The Science behind The
Biggest Loser's Failure*. ZoneDiet.

204. Pitney, N. (2009, November 25). *Biggest Loser: Contestants Admit
Dangerous Practices, Can't Speak Out*. The Huffington Post.

205. Kolata, G. (2016, May 2). *After "The Biggest Loser," Their Bodies Fought
to Regain Weight*. The New York Times. https://www.nytimes.com/
2016/05/02/health/biggest-loser-weight-loss.html

206. National Eating Disorders Association. (n.d.). *Anorexia Nervosa*. NEDA.
https://www.nationaleatingdisorders.org/anorexia-nervosa/

207. Jackson-Cannady, A. (2013, December 17). *Master Your
Metabolism*. WebMD. https://www.webmd.com/diet/a-z/master-
your-metabolism-diet

208. American Heart Association. (2021). *How Much Physical Activity Do
You Need?* https://www.heart.org/en/healthy-living/fitness/fitness-
basics/aha-recs-for-physical-activity-infographic

209. Ramos, T. (2024, July 15). *Sam Sulek's Workout to Grow 20-Inch Arms*. Generation Iron Fitness & Strength Sports Network. https://generationiron.com/sam-sulek-arm-workout/

210 Bagchi, S. (2024, March 21). *21-Y.O. Sam Sulek Finally Breaks Silence about His Competitive Future in Bodybuilding*. EssentiallySports. https://www.essentiallysports.com/bodybuilding-news-twenty-one-y-o-sam-sulek-finally-breaks-silence-about-his-competitive-future-in-bodybuilding/

211. Waehner, P. (2021). *Everything You Need to Know about Muscle Failure*. Verywell Fit. https://www.verywellfit.com/muscle-failure-1231090

212. Sweatt, L. (2023, November 21). *Sam Sulek Breaks Every YouTube Rule, Still Goes Insanely Viral*. VidIQ. https://vidiq.com/blog/post/sam-sulek-breaks-youtube-rules-goes-viral/

213. DeAngelis, T. (2024, April 1). *Teens Are Spending Nearly 5 Hours Daily on Social Media: Here Are the Mental Health Outcomes*. American Psychological Association. https://www.apa.org/monitor/2024/04/teen-social-use-mental-health

214. O'Neill, N. (2023, February 23). *Less Social Media Improves Teens' Body Image: Study*. New York Post. https://nypost.com/2023/02/23/less-social-media-improves-teens-body-image-study/

215. Gaddis, J. (2020, September 21). *The Big Business of School Meals*. PDK International. https://kappanonline.org/big-business-school-meals-food-service-gaddis/

216. Mensendiek, H. (2023, October 5). *Report: Nearly Half of Dietary Guidelines Advisory Committee Have Conflicts of Interest*. U.S. Right to Know. https://usrtk.org/investigations/dietary-guidelines-advisory-committee-conflicts/

217. Mensendiek, H., Morrison, B., Pampalone, T., Malkan, S., & Ruskin, G. (n.d.). *Full Disclosure Assessing Conflicts of Interest of the 2025 Dietary Guidelines Advisory Committee*. https://usrtk.org/wp-content/uploads/dietary-guidelines-advisory-committee-conflicts-2023.pdf

218. StockAnalysis. (2014). *Tyson Foods Revenue 2014-2024*. Stock Analysis. https://stockanalysis.com/stocks/tsn/revenue/

219. StockAnalysis. (2025). *Sodexo (SDXOF) Stock Price & Overview*. StockAnalysis. https://stockanalysis.com/quote/otc/SDXOF/

220. United States Department of Agriculture. (2024, June 11). *National School Lunch Program Factsheet | Food and Nutrition Service*. https://www.fns.usda.gov/nslp/factsheet

221. School Nutrition Association. (n.d.). *School Meal Statistics - School Nutrition Association.* https://schoolnutrition.org/about-school-meals/school-meal-statistics/#scheduling

222. FoodCorps. (2025, June 10). *The Policy Brief: 2025 State Policy Updates FoodCorps.* https://foodcorps.org/blog-policy-2025-state-updates/

223. Sole-Smith, V. (2021, September 21). *Please Stop Romanticizing Your Child's Lunchbox.* Substack.com; Burnt Toast by Virginia Sole-Smith. https://virginiasolesmith.substack.com/p/please-stop-romanticizing-your-childs

224. Algar, S. (2021, August 27). *Wisconsin School Board Blasted for Saying Kids Might Get "Spoiled" by Free Lunch.* New York Post. https://nypost.com/2021/08/27/wisconsin-school-board-member-says-kids-might-get-spoiled-by-free-lunch/

225. Terrell, J., host. "The Paradox of Plenty Amid Hunger" Left Over, LWC Studios, March 15, 2023. LeftOverPod.com

226. Spence, S. M. (2022). *Shana Minei Spence, MS, RDN, CDN (@ thenutritiontea) on Threads.* Threads. https://www.threads.com/@thenutritiontea/post/Cuhf9x0LfuV

227. Williams-Forson, P. A. (2022). *Eating While Black.* UNC Press Books.

228. UCONN Rudd Center. (2020, April 20). *Measuring Student & School Wellness.* https://uconnruddcenter.org/research/schools/school-wellness/

229. Pickens, A. L. (n.d.). *Fatphobia at Work: How to Recognize It & End It.* InHerSight. https://www.inhersight.com/blog/allyship/fatphobia

230. U.S. Department of Agriculture. (2000). *Local School Wellness Policy.* USDA; Food and Nutrition Service. https://www.fns.usda.gov/tn/local-school-wellness-policy

231. Tufts University. (2021, April 6). *Study Finds Americans Eat Food of Mostly Poor Nutritional Quality – Except at School.* Tufts Now. https://now.tufts.edu/news-releases/study-finds-americans-eat-food-mostly-poor-nutritional-quality-except-school

232. Government Accountability Office. (2023). *School Meals: USDA Should Address Challenges in Its "Foods in Schools" Program.* U.S. GAO. https://www.gao.gov/products/gao-23-105697

233. Open Secrets. (2025). *Food & Beverage Lobbying Profile.* OpenSecrets. https://www.opensecrets.org/federal-lobbying/industries/summary?cycle=2024&id=N01

234. Open Secrets. (2024). *Food & Beverage Lobbying Profile.* OpenSecrets. https://www.opensecrets.org/federal-lobbying/industries/summary?cycle=2024&id=N01

235. Pinson, N. (2022, November 17). *Soda Contracts.* Rethinking Schools. https://rethinkingschools.org/articles/soda-contracts-who-really-benefits/

236. Terrell, J., host. "Their Job Is Not to Make Kids Healthier" Left Over, LWC Studios, March 15, 2023. LeftOverPod.com

237. Andersen, K. (Director). (2017). *What the Health.* Netflix.

238. The National Agricultural Law Center. (n.d.). *Checkoff Programs - National Agricultural Law Center.* https://nationalaglawcenter.org/research-by-topic/checkoff-programs/

239. Gonzales, M. (2024, January 6). *Confronting Weight Bias.* https://www.shrm.org/topics-tools/news/all-things-work/confronting-weight-bias

240. United States Department of Agriculture. (2024a). *Comparison Chart of the 2023 Proposed and 2024 Final Rule Requirements for School Meal Programs | Food and Nutrition Service.* USDA Food and Nutrition Service. https://www.fns.usda.gov/cn/school-nutrition-standards-updates/rule-comparison-chart

241. Magnus, A., & Stasio, F. (2018, May 29). *A Big Look at Big Hog In North Carolina.* WUNC. https://www.wunc.org/business-economy/2018-05-29/a-big-look-at-big-hog-in-north-carolina

242. NCGE. (2014). *North Carolina in the Global Economy: Hog Farming.* https://ncglobaleconomy.com/hog/overview.shtml

243. Oglesby, C. (2021, May 17). *Hurricane Season Spurs Hog Waste Worries in North Carolina.* Environmental Health News. https://www.ehn.org/north-carolina-hurricanes-hog-farms-2652972415.html

244. Baars, S. (2025, February 16). *North Carolina's Hog Problem.* Southern Environmental Law Center. https://www.selc.org/news/the-sinister-hog-industry-of-eastern-north-carolina/

245. Berger, J. (2022, April 1). *How Black North Carolinians Pay the Price for the World's Cheap Bacon.* Vox. https://www.vox.com/future-perfect/23003487/north-carolina-hog-pork-bacon-farms-environmental-racism-black-residents-pollution-meat-industry

246. Jansen, D. (2022, October 4). *Teaching While Fat.* This Magazine. https://this.org/2022/10/04/teaching-while-fat/

247. Ramirez, M. (2025, January 23). *Trump's Executive Orders Take Aim at Environmental Justice Measures: What It Means*. USA TODAY. https://www.usatoday.com/story/news/nation/2025/01/22/environmental-justice-trump-revokes-advances-by-clinton-biden/77886090007/

248. The White House. (2025, January 20). *Ending Radical and Wasteful Government DEI Programs and Preferencing*. The White House. https://www.whitehouse.gov/presidential-actions/2025/01/ending-radical-and-wasteful-government-dei-programs-and-preferencing/

249. Jalonick, M. (2011, November 15). *Pizza Is a Vegetable? Congress Says Yes*. NBC News. https://www.nbcnews.com/health/health-news/pizza-vegetable-congress-says-yes-flna1C9453097

250. Nwuba, C. (2025). *Food Is NOT Just about Calories: It Can Be Culture, Nourishment, Self-Care, Love, Fun, Hope and Friendship—All in One*. X (Formerly Twitter). https://x.com/drchuks_/status/1593671520974512140

251. Secretary for Health and Human Services. (2025, April 22). *HHS, FDA to Phase Out Petroleum-Based Synthetic Dyes in Nation's Food Supply*. The U.S. Department of Health and Human Services. https://www.hhs.gov/press-room/hhs-fda-food-dyes-food.html

252 Todd, R. (2025, June 9). *Food Safety Expert Discusses Science Behind FDA's Changes to Food Dye Rules*. WVTF. https://www.wvtf.org/news/2025-06-09/food-safety-expert-discusses-science-behind-fdas-changes-to-food-dye-rules

253. PBS NewsHour. (2025). Watch: RFK Jr. and West Virginia Gov. Morrisey Make Announcements on Food Dye, Proposed SNAP Changes. *YouTube*. https://www.youtube.com/watch?v=jl3LDq5HL-8

254. Yandell, K. (2025, April 16). *Hits and Misses in RFK Jr.'s Comments on Food Dyes*. FactCheck.org. https://www.factcheck.org/2025/04/hits-and-misses-in-rfk-jr-s-comments-on-food-dyes/

255. The New York Post. (2022). Tiktok.com; TikTok. https://www.tiktok.com/@nypost/video/7486948989439315242?_r=1&_t=ZP-8v4Kds9TLCw

256. Flam, C. (2025). *RFK Jr. Mercilessly Fat Shames West Virginia Governor at Live Joint Appearance*. People.com. https://people.com/rfk-jr-mercilessly-fat-shames-west-virginia-governor-at-live-joint-appearance-11705534

257. Marling, S. (2025, March 22). *Full Plates to Paperwork: Federal Cuts to Free Lunch Program Could Burden WV Schools*. Charleston Gazette-Mail. https://www.wvgazettemail.com/news/education/full-plates-to-paperwork-federal-cuts-to-free-lunch-program-could-burden-wv-schools/article_274f87a4-0476-11f0-98f9-d7283ba97b16.html

258. United States Senate Committee on Agriculture, Nutrition and Forestry. (2025, May 29). *CBO Confirms: Millions of Food Insecure Americans Will See Higher Food Costs due to Congressional Republicans' SNAP Cuts*. The United States Senate Committee on Agriculture, Nutrition & Forestry. https://www.agriculture.senate.gov/newsroom/dem/press/release/cbo-confirms-millions-of-food-insecure-americans-will-see-higher-food-costs-due-to-congressional-republicans-snap-cuts

259. Newman, J. (2025). *RFK Jr. Pledges No Twinkie Ban*. The Wall Street Journal. https://www.wsj.com/livecoverage/trump-cabinet-confirmation-hearings/card/rfk-jr-pledges-no-twinkie-ban-TTKuaQRpWjixqbHAqF2h?gaa_at=eafs&gaa_n=ASWzDAi3PYWSEgp7sUYYeF2JlhY5hZha9sQr3_CmQVD5CFxyCU3ECRhCuGs_qrJysro%3D&gaa_ts=6850545f&gaa_sig=P_LiHcajJ23lkgpfwvY_Mvgn1s-g7i1YyPlkbHobnQAsob5Ni-diK6lZNZiJt32agFpudEbeaWO06C433rFlgA%3D%3D

260. Kolata, G. (2025, April 7). *As RFK Jr. Champions Chronic Disease Prevention, Key Research Is Cut*. The New York Times. https://www.nytimes.com/2025/04/07/health/rfk-hhs-diabetes-obesity-disease.html

261. Sole-Smith, V. (2025, April 29). *Fat Moms Don't Cause Autism*. Burnt Toast by Virginia Sole-Smith. https://virginiasolesmith.substack.com/p/fat-moms-dont-cause-autism

262. Suren, P., Gunnes, N., Roth, C., et al. (2014). Parental Obesity and Risk of Autism Spectrum Disorder. *Pediatrics*, *133*(5), e1128–e1138. https://doi.org/10.1542/peds.2013-3664

263. Yandell, K. (2023, August 10). *What RFK Jr. Gets Wrong about Autism*. FactCheck.org. https://www.factcheck.org/2023/08/scicheck-what-rfk-jr-gets-wrong-about-autism/

264. Demirjian, K., Blum, D., & Ghorayshi, A. (2025, April 16). *RFK Jr. Calls Autism "Preventable," Drawing Ire from Researchers*. The New York Times. https://www.nytimes.com/2025/04/16/us/politics/rfk-jr-autism.html?unlocked_article_code=1.B08.G5mn.jt_3PF_S329D&smid=url-share

265. Simmons-Duffin, S. (2025, June 8). *RFK Jr. Says Americans Were Healthier When His Uncle Was President: Is He Right?* NPR. https://www.npr.org/2025/06/06/nx-s1-5399616/rfk-jr-life-expectancy-chronic-disease-maha

266. Autism Science Foundation. (2025, April 16). *RFK Disputes Results of CDC Autism Prevalence Study Citing "Common Sense" but No Actual Science*. Autism Science Foundation - Supporting and Sharing Autism Research to Improve the Real Lives of Real People. https://autismsciencefoundation.org/press_releases/statement-prevalence-study/

267. Kennedy, R. F. (2024). *End the Chronic Disease Epidemic*. Kennedy24. https://web.archive.org/web/20240709185952/https://www.kennedy24.com/end-chronic-disease

268. Skinner, A. (2024, August 23). *RFK Jr. Calls Out Obese Americans: "They Were Sent to the Circus."* Newsweek. https://www.newsweek.com/rfk-jr-calls-out-obese-americans-sent-circus-1943788

269. Kiger, P. J. (2023, May 2). *The Health Problems JFK Hid from the Public*. HISTORY. https://www.history.com/articles/the-health-problems-jfk-hid-from-the-public

270. Sole-Smith, V. (2023, May 23). *Michelle Obama Is Not Coming to Save Us*. Burnt Toast by Virginia Sole-Smith. https://virginiasolesmith.substack.com/p/michelle-obama-is-not-coming-to-save-us

271. Halpert, M. (2025, January 28). *Weight-loss Drugs Could Set Up Clash Between RFK Jr and Aides*. BBC. https://www.bbc.com/news/articles/cvg84zelwepo

272. Bakst, D. (2019). *Michelle Obama Shouldn't Decide What Your Child Eats*. The Heritage Foundation. https://www.heritage.org/education/commentary/michelle-obama-shouldnt-decide-what-your-child-eats

273. Bakst, D. (2014, June 24). *Why Michelle Obama Is Wrong on School Lunches*. The Heritage Foundation. https://www.heritage.org/public-health/commentary/why-michelle-obama-wrong-school-lunches

274. Let's Move! (2010). *The Partnership for a Healthier America*. Let's Move! https://letsmove.obamawhitehouse.archives.gov/partnership-healthier-america

275. Hardee, C. (2020, April 20). *Food Marketing in Schools | School Nutrition.* UConn Rudd Center. https://uconnruddcenter.org/research/schools/marketing/

276. Leonard, A. (2011). *The Story of Stuff: How Our Obsession with Stuff Is Trashing the Planet, Our Communities, and Our Health-and a Vision for Change.* Free Press.

277. Hanson, O. (2021). *PSA for Parents, Teachers, and Coaches: That Food Being Labeled as "Bad," "Junk," or "Unhealthy" Might Be One of the Few Safe Foods for a Child with an Eating Disorder or Other Medical Condition.* https://x.com/OonaHanson/status/1469759305121349632

278. Equip Health. (n.d.). *What Is ARFID (Avoidant Restrictive Food Intake Disorder)?* https://equip.health/conditions/arfid

279. Boehm, R., Read, M., Henderson, K. E., & Schwartz, M. B. (2019). Removing Competitive Foods v. Nudging and Marketing School Meals: A Pilot Study in High-school Cafeterias. *Public Health Nutrition, 23*(2), 366–373. https://doi.org/10.1017/s136898001900329x

280. FDA. (2023, October 17). *Generally Recognized as Safe (GRAS).* U.S. Food and Drug Administration. https://www.fda.gov/food/food-ingredients-packaging/generally-recognized-safe-gras

281. The White House. (2012). *Race to the Top.* The White House. https://obamawhitehouse.archives.gov/issues/education/k-12/race-to-the-top

282. Nestle, M. (2023, May 10). *PLEZi: Better for Kids? Healthier?* Food Politics by Marion Nestle. https://www.foodpolitics.com/2023/05/plezi-healthier-for-kids-maybe-but-healthy/

283. FoodCorps. (2023, February 13). *Nourishing Futures™.* https://foodcorps.org/nourishing-futures/

284. FoodCorps. (2020). *Sugar Showdown.* https://foodcorps.org/wp-content/uploads/2018/07/Grade-5-Sugar-Showdown-1.pdf

285. Drayer, L. (2019, April 18). *Does Sugar Make Kids Hyper? That's Largely a Myth.* CNN. https://www.cnn.com/2019/04/18/health/sugar-hyper-myth-food-drayer/index.html

286. Rosenkranz, R., Warner, N., Yarrow, L., & Rosenkranz, S. (2021). *Use of Food Rewards in Education: Time to De-implement this Practice?* https://schoolnutrition.org/journal/fall-2021-use-of-food-rewards-in-education-time-to-de-implement-this-practice/

287. Paris, D., & Alim, H. S. (2017). *Culturally Sustaining Pedagogies: Teaching and Learning for Justice in a Changing World*. Teachers College Press.

288. USDA. (2014, May 20). *Fact Sheet: Healthy, Hunger-Free Kids Act School Meals Implementation*. USDA. https://www.usda.gov/about-usda/news/press-releases/2014/05/20/fact-sheet-healthy-hunger-free-kids-act-school-meals-implementation

289. Ansel, K., & Ellis, E. (2022, June 29). *Sugar: Does It Really Cause Hyperactivity?* eatright. https://www.eatright.org/health/wellness/healthful-habits/sugar-does-it-really-cause-hyperactivity

290. WebMD Archives. (n.d.). *Busting the Sugar-Hyperactivity Myth*. WebMD. https://www.webmd.com/parenting/features/busting-sugar-hyperactivity-myth

291. Arnold, T. (2024, July 17). *Dr. Taylor Arnold • Kid Nutrition Expert (Ph D, RDN) on Instagram: "I'm not opposed to stuff like removing candy and soda from vending machines or not allowing candy as classroom rewards. But I do not like a grams of sugar limit per serving on foods. 💬 What do you think? #healthyrelationshipwithfood #intuitiveeating #pickyeater #fussyeater #adhdkids #adhdnutrition #gentleparenting #respectfulparenting #cyclebreaker #teachersoftiktok."* Instagram. https://www.instagram.com/p/C9ie-Y5yJ0E/

292. King County Green Schools Program. (2020). *Longer Lunch Periods in K-12 Schools: Research Summary with References*. https://your.kingcounty.gov/dnrp/library/solid-waste/programs/green-schools/food-waste-longer-seated-lunch-periods.pdf

293. Prothero, A. (2023, April 25). *Are Lunch Periods Too Short? Some States Want to Give Kids More Time to Eat*. Education Week. https://www.edweek.org/leadership/are-lunch-periods-too-short-some-states-want-to-give-kids-more-time-to-eat/2023/04

294. Center for Disease Control. (2019, July 29). *Making Time for School Lunch*. CDC. https://www.cdc.gov/healthyschools/nutrition/school_lunch.htm

295. Gvozdas, S. (2018). *Longer Lunch, More Options*. Baltimore Sun. https://www.baltimoresun.com/news/bs-xpm-2008-02-03-0802010313-story.html

296. Scholastic Choices. (2017). Do Teens Need Recess? *Scholastic Choices*.

297. Tatum, B. D. (2017). *"Why Are All the Black Kids Sitting Together in the Cafeteria?": And Other Conversations about Race*. Basic Books. (Original work published 1997)

298. Blake, S. (2023, December 6). *Weight Discrimination Laws Spread to More States*. Newsweek. https://www.newsweek.com/anti-size-discrimination-laws-states-companies-policies-1849823

299. Stop Bullying. (2018, November 2). *Preventing Weight-Based Bullying*. StopBullying.gov. https://www.stopbullying.gov/blog/2018/11/05/preventing-weight-based-bullying

300. Chen, G. (2012, May 7). *Longer Lunches, Smarter Students? The Controversy of 10 Minute or 1 Hour Lunch Periods*. Public School Review. https://www.publicschoolreview.com/blog/longer-lunches-smarter-students-the-controversy-of-10-minute-or-1-hour-lunch-periods

301. Mader, J. (2022, May 12). *Recess Guidelines Vary Greatly from State to State*. The Hechinger Report. https://hechingerreport.org/kids-access-to-recess-varies-greatly/

302. Suzuki, K. (2024, January 30). *For the First Time, California Law Will Protect Students' Right to Recess*. KPBS Public Media. https://www.kpbs.org/news/health/2024/01/30/for-the-first-time-california-law-will-protect-students-right-to-recess

303. Sole-Smith, V. (2023a, August 8). *When Diet Culture Comes to Soccer Practice*. Substack; Burnt Toast by Virginia Sole Smith. https://virginiasolesmith.substack.com/p/when-diet-culture-shows-up-at-soccer

304. Sole-Smith, V. (2023, September 28). *The Fat Theater Kids Survival Guide*. Substack.com; Burnt Toast by Virginia Sole-Smith. https://virginiasolesmith.substack.com/p/fat-theater-kids

305. NYCLU. (2024, May 15). *Court Strikes Down Nassau County Anti-Trans Sports Ban*. NYCLU. https://www.nyclu.org/press-release/court-strikes-down-nassau-county-anti-trans-sports-ban

306. Lewis, R. C. (2025, May 6). *Senate Committee Advances GOP Anti-trans Bill*. City & State New York. https://www.cityandstateny.com/policy/2025/05/senate-committee-advances-gop-anti-trans-bill/405093/

307. McGregor, K., McKenna, J. L., Barrera, E. P., Williams, C. R., Hartman-Munick, S. M., & Guss, C. E. (2023). Disordered Eating and Considerations for the Transgender Community: A Review of the Literature and Clinical Guidance for Assessment and Treatment.

Journal of Eating Disorders, 11(1). https://doi.org/10.1186/s40337-023-00793-0

308. The White House. (2025b, February 5). *Keeping Men Out of Women's Sports*. The White House. https://www.whitehouse.gov/presidential-actions/2025/02/keeping-men-out-of-womens-sports/

309. Gregory, S. (2023, November 2). *Caster Semenya Isn't Just Fighting for Herself*. TIME. https://time.com/6330414/caster-semenya-race-to-be-myself-interview/

310. Power, S. (2024, August 23). *JK Rowling Breaks Silence after Lawsuit, Renews Attack on Imane Khelif*. Newsweek. https://www.newsweek.com/jk-rowling-imane-khelif-lawsuit-twitter-1943502

311. Murphy, B. (2024, August 9). *Imane Khelif Condition, Explained: Fact-checking the XY Chromosome at Center of Gender Eligibility Controversy*. The Sporting News. https://www.sportingnews.com/us/olympics/news/imane-khelif-condition-explained-gender-fact-check/51994b8a2e23e7b423782f7a

312. Advisor. (2024, October 28). *The Controversy of Imane Khelif*. The Spectator. https://spectator.mcpherson.edu/2024/10/the-controversy-of-imane-khelif/

313. Stubbs, R. (2019, October 15). *For High School Offensive Linemen, Fat-Shaming and Health Risks Come with the Territory*. The Washington Post. https://www.washingtonpost.com/sports/2019/10/15/high-school-offensive-linemen-fat-shaming-health-risks-come-with-territory/

314. Guzdek, G. (Ed.). (2022, February 23). *Diet Culture Is Ruining Female Athletes*. Hartford Courant. https://www.courant.com/2022/02/23/gabby-guzdek-diet-culture-is-ruining-female-athletes/

315. Shaffer, L. (2023, March 20). *Wrestling with Diet Culture: How High School Sports Contributed to My Eating Disorder*. Oregon Live. https://www.oregonlive.com/education/2023/03/wrestling-with-diet-culture-how-high-school-sports-contributed-to-my-eating-disorder.html

316. Ronshaugen, N., Moffatt, K., & Koontz, J. (2022, October 5). *Rules in Place to Guard against Weight Cutting in Wrestling*. NFHS. https://www.nfhs.org/articles/rules-in-place-to-guard-against-weight-cutting-in-wrestling/

317. Bailey, M. (2023, March 1). *Athletes and Disordered Eating: Who Is at Risk and How to Get Help*. MultiCare Vitals. https://www.multicare.

org/vitals/athletes-and-disordered-eating-who-is-at-risk-and-how-to-get-help/

318. USA Triathlon. (2023, October 4). *Six Things to Avoid When Talking to Athletes about Sports Nutrition.* https://www.usatriathlon.org/articles/features/six-things-to-avoid-when-talking-to-athletes-about-sports-nutrition

319. Girl Scouts USA. (n.d.). *Girl Scout Alumnae by the Numbers.* https://www.girlscouts.org/content/dam/girlscouts-gsusa/forms-and-documents/about-girl-scouts/research/gs-alumnae-by-the-numbers.pdf

320. Hanson, O. (2025, January 30). *People Can't Stop Being Jerks to Girl Scouts.* Parenting Without Diet Culture. https://oonahanson.substack.com/p/people-cant-stop-being-jerks-to-girl

321. Moore, L. (2022, February 24). *Girl Scout Cookie Sellers as Young as 5 Are Being Harassed for Selling Unhealthy Food and a Conspiracy Theory about Cookie Money Funding Abortion.* Business Insider. https://www.businessinsider.com/girl-scout-cookies-harassment-planned-parenthood-abortion-unhealthy-palm-oil-2022-2

322. Hurley, K. (2023, February 8). *Don't Serve Girl Scout Cookies with a Side of Shame.* CNN. https://www.cnn.com/2023/02/08/health/girl-scout-cookies-body-image-wellness

323. Smith, J. D. (2024, February 2). *Watching My Daughter Sell Girl Scout Cookies Made Me Realize It's Time to Stop Talking about Weight and Diet around Kids.* Yahoo!Life; Yahoo! https://www.yahoo.com/lifestyle/watching-my-daughter-sell-girl-scout-cookies-made-me-realize-its-time-to-stop-talking-about-weight-and-diet-around-kids-164149509.html?guce_referrer=aHR0cHM6Ly93d3cuZ29vZ2xlLmNvbS8&guce_referrer_sig=AQAAACTF0WXEtDNvevdti2q0OP0BlGY02L26YJ6pzUZUflF_hA5tDO2VnuZlff6liKG6ywia06KMkmZWwrWnqobJnZKG8bTuhsouZ0_TxzMSb-ilbBQvbvQinxaqdD8VQ_zlbrmZef9Q6MQyWrEp05PMsl3_yab6xs6QMWP9eZlCA6L&guccounter=2

324. U.S. Department of Defense. (2023). *U.S. Army JROTC New Pamphlet.* https://www.usarmyjrotc.com/wp-content/uploads/2023/03/New-JROTC-Brochure-2023.pdf

325. Aina Marzia. (2022, September 6). *How Counter-Recruiters Take on the U.S. Military.* YES! Magazine. https://www.yesmagazine.org/

social-justice/2022/09/06/military-recruitment-youth-of-color%EF%BF%BC

326. Beynon, S. (2023, December 20). *Military Focusing on JROTC Programs as Chances to Paint Picture of Service to Gen Z Dwindle.* Military.com. https://www.military.com/daily-news/2023/12/19/military-focusing-jrotc-programs-chances-paint-picture-of-service-gen-z-dwindle.html

327. Kheel, R. (2022, November 16). *60 Junior ROTC Instructors Accused of Sexual Misconduct in Past Five Years, Investigation Finds.* Military.com. https://www.military.com/daily-news/2022/11/16/60-junior-rotc-instructors-accused-of-sexual-misconduct-past-five-years-investigation-finds.html

328. Rice, C. E. (2024, November 21). *Less Is More: Turning Overweight Recruits into Warriors.* AUSA. https://www.ausa.org/articles/less-more-turning-overweight-recruits-warriors

329. Goldman, C., Schweig, J., Buenaventura, M., & Wright, C. (2017). *Geographic and Demographic Representativeness of Junior Reserve Officer Training Corps.* The RAND Corporation. https://www.rand.org/content/dam/rand/pubs/research_reports/RR1700/RR1712/RAND_RR1712.pdf

330. Camacho, R. (2022, April 18). *Marginalized Students Pay the Price of Military Recruitment Efforts.* Prism. https://prismreports.org/2022/04/18/marginalized-students-military-recruitment/

331 Stark, S. (2023, January 24). *Why Is It Still Legal to Fire Someone for Being Fat?* WBEZ Chicago. https://www.wbez.org/reset-with-sasha-ann-simons/2023/01/24/why-is-it-still-legal-to-fire-someone-for-being-fat

332. Sisson, S. B., Malek-Lasater, A., Ford, T. G., Horm, D., & Kwon, K.-A. (2023). Predictors of Overweight and Obesity in Early Care and Education Teachers during COVID-19. *International Journal of Environmental Research and Public Health, 20*(3), 2763. https://doi.org/10.3390/ijerph20032763

333. Parker, E. A., Feinberg, T. M., Lane, H. G., Deitch, R., Zemanick, A., Saksvig, B. I., Turner, L., & Hager, E. R. (2020). Diet Quality of Elementary and Middle School Teachers Is Associated with Healthier Nutrition-Related Classroom Practices. *Preventive Medicine Reports, 18*, 101087. https://doi.org/10.1016/j.pmedr.2020.101087

334. Klein, A. (2021, December 6). *1,500 Decisions a Day (At Least!): How Teachers Cope with a Dizzying Array of Questions*. Education Week. https://www.edweek.org/teaching-learning/1-500-decisions-a-day-at-least-how-teachers-cope-with-a-dizzying-array-of-questions/2021/12

335. Mitchell-Rose, H. (2023, March 27). *On Being a Fat Preschool Teacher*. Great Fat-Itude! https://www.greatfatitude.com/blog/on-being-a-fat-preschool-teacher

336. Cait O'Connor. (2024, July 26). *The Right to Remain Seated*. Cait's Substack. https://substack.com/home/post/p-146847723

337. Griffiths, B. (2022). *Teacher Positioning in the Classroom*. TeachingEnglish. https://www.teachingenglish.org.uk/professional-development/teachers/managing-lesson/articles/teacher-positioning-classroom

338. Bevan, S. (2019, January 21). *Half of Employers Say They Are Less Inclined to Recruit Obese Candidates – It's Not OK*. The Conversation. https://theconversation.com/half-of-employers-say-they-are-less-inclined-to-recruit-obese-candidates-its-not-ok-109821

339. Abrahams Brosbe, R. (2022). *Fatphobia Showed Up in My Classroom*. Rethinking Schools. https://rethinkingschools.org/articles/fatphobia-showed-up-in-my-classroom/

340. Duffie, M. (2022, August 6). *How to Combat Anti-Fatness in the Workplace*. Linkedin. https://www.linkedin.com/pulse/how-combat-anti-fatness-workplace-michelle-duffie

341. Fay, C., & Sole-Smith, V. (2025, January 9). *You Can Count Your Protein and Still Be Nice to Fat People*. Burnt Toast by Virginia Sole-Smith. https://virginiasolesmith.substack.com/p/you-can-count-your-protein-and-still-be-nice-to-fat-people?utm_source=%2Finbox%2Fpaid&utm_medium=reader2

342. Gordon, A. (2020b, August 27). *Talking about Our Body Image Issues Can Be Harmful: That's Why We Should Ask for Consent First*. SELF. https://www.self.com/story/body-talk-consent

343. Harrison, C. (2019, May 13). *Why Fatphobia Hurts All of Us with Sofie Hagen* (No. 195) [Podcast]. Apple Podcast.

344. Gordon, A. (2020c, September 1). *Please Don't Bring Up "Skinny Shaming" When We Talk about Fat Shaming*. SELF. https://www.self.com/story/skinny-shaming

345. Willett, W., Wood, M., & Childs, D. (2014). *Thinfluence: Thin-flu-ence (noun) the Powerful and Surprising Effect Friends, Family, Work, and Environment Have on Weight*. Rodale.

346. Oxford Languages. (n.d.). *Concern Troll Definition*. https://tinyurl.com/4rv7339v

347. Gordon, A. (2021, August 24). *Weight-Focused "Workplace Wellness" Programs Drive Stigma and Inequity—It's Time to End Them*. SELF. https://www.self.com/story/weight-workplace-wellness

348. Gordon, A. (2020a, August 7). *We Have to Stop Thinking of Being "Healthy" as Being Morally Better*. SELF. https://www.self.com/story/healthism

349. Ellin, A. (2015, September 16). *How Obamacare Allows Companies to Punish Fat Employees*. Observer. https://observer.com/2015/09/unwell-how-the-affordable-care-act-lets-companies-punish-fat-employees/

350. Dively, C. (2024). *Staff Members Participate in Biggest Loser Competition*. Mountain Echo. https://aahsmountainecho.com/32646/news/staff-members-participate-in-biggest-loser-competition/

351. Dearborn Schools. (2016). *Official Rules for the "Biggest Loser" Contest Sponsored by DSEHP for Dearborn Public Schools*. https://dearbornschools.org/stout/wp-content/uploads/sites/50/2016/01/DSEHP-Biggest-Loser-Contest-Official-Rules.pdf

352. Ham, A. (2025). *Biggest Loser*. Teachers Pay Teachers. https://www.teacherspayteachers.com/browse?search=biggest%20loser

353. Lee, K. M., Hunger, J. M., & Tomiyama, A. J. (2021). Weight Stigma and Health Behaviors: Evidence from the Eating in America Study. *International Journal of Obesity*, *45*(7). https://doi.org/10.1038/s41366-021-00814-5

354. Hagy, P. (2023). *From Bezos and Zuckerberg Getting Buff to the Celebrity Ozempic Craze, "Fatphobia" in the Workplace Is More Rampant Than Ever*. Fortune Well. https://fortune.com/well/2023/08/01/fatphobia-obesity-weight-loss-discrimination-workplace-ozempic-zuckerberg-bezos-musk/

355. Petrilli, M. J. (2024). *U.S. Schools' Next Big Problem: The Cost of Teacher Obesity*. The Thomas B. Fordham Institute. https://fordhaminstitute.org/ohio/commentary/us-schools-next-big-problem-cost-teacher-obesity

For Product Safety Concerns and Information please contact our EU
representative GPSR@taylorandfrancis.com
Taylor & Francis Verlag GmbH, Kaufingerstraße 24, 80331 München, Germany